The Myths of Nutrition and Fitness

Anthony A. Goodman, M.D., F.A.C.S.

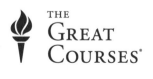

THE
GREAT
COURSES

PUBLISHED BY:

THE GREAT COURSES
Corporate Headquarters
4840 Westfields Boulevard, Suite 500
Chantilly, Virginia 20151-2299
Phone: 1-800-832-2412
Fax: 703-378-3819
www.thegreatcourses.com

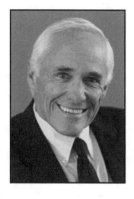

Anthony A. Goodman, M.D., F.A.C.S.
Adjunct Professor of Medicine
Montana State University

Professor Anthony A. Goodman received his B.A. from Harvard College and his M.D. from Cornell Medical College. He trained as a surgical intern and resident at the University of Michigan Medical Center in Ann Arbor and completed his surgical training and served as chief resident at the Harvard Surgical Service of Boston City Hospital, New England Deaconess Hospital, Lahey Clinic, and Cambridge City Hospital.

Dr. Goodman served as a surgeon on the hospital ship for Project HOPE and served with the U.S. Army Medical Corps from 1971 to 1973. From 1973 to 1992, he was a general surgeon, specializing in the surgical treatment of cancer, and was Clinical Associate Professor of Surgery at the University of Miami School of Medicine. In 1991, he was Visiting Professor of Surgery at the Christchurch Clinical School of Medicine in Christchurch, New Zealand.

Dr. Goodman has served as an examiner for the American Board of Surgery. He is a Fellow of the American College of Surgeons and a Diplomate of the American Board of Surgery. He has been a member of the American Society of Colon and Rectal Surgeons and the British Association of Surgical Oncology. He was the founder of the Broward Surgical Society. He has published numerous papers on both clinical and experimental surgery.

At present, Dr. Goodman is Adjunct Professor of Medicine in the WWAMI Medical Sciences Program at Montana State University, where he teaches gross anatomy, and Affiliate Professor in the Department of Biological Structure at the University of Washington School of Medicine.

Dr. Goodman is also the author of a work of historical fiction, *The Shadow of God: A Novel of War and Faith* (Sourcebooks Landmark, 2002). ■

ACKNOWLEDGMENTS

In researching and creating these lectures I was most fortunate to have the guidance and wisdom of a cadre of amazing people, especially those much, much younger than I. This insightful group included my adult children, Katie Goodman and Cameron Goodman, as well as their partners Soren Kisiel and Liora Ziv, along with Nathan Ziv and Abbey Bier-Ziv. Many hours were spent discussing ideas that mattered as they are all very fit and quite interested in nutrition. My thanks and appreciation to you all.

Once again I also want to acknowledge the input and guidance from my wife, Maribeth Goodman, who was instrumental in the creation of these lectures. Fitness and nutrition are lifelong passions for us both and it was great fun to co-create this series with her for The Great Courses.

A percentage of the professor royalties from this course will be donated to: Water For People – www.waterforpeople.org. ■

Table of Contents

The Myths of Nutrition and Fitness

Scope:

We have to face the facts: In our quest for health and longevity there is no single quick fix and there are factors beyond our control, such as genetic predispositions. But even if nothing can guarantee a long and healthy life, when it comes to increasing our odds of attaining this desirable goal, nothing beats the combination of a well balanced diet of fresh whole foods together with lifelong vigorous body movement. There are hundreds of healthy combinations of whole foods, and countless ways to move your body that will all pay you enormous benefits.

This course goes beyond simplistic edicts of loading up on carbohydrates before running and staying hydrated to crack the myths of food and fitness. How do different food groups affect our bodies depending on the activity—from biking and running to hiking and basketball? What should we eat, drink, and avoid before, during, and after our workouts? What activities with the appropriate nutrition plans will serve us in a meaningful way? What are the keys to eating and drinking in ways that best support our fitness and athletic routines? Each lecture addre198sses some of the myths and realities concerning the relationship between nutrition and fitness.

Throughout this series we will look at some of the science behind the relationships between dietary practices and athletics, exercise, sports, and just overall fitness. These lectures provide you with some of the tools you will need to examine the pros and cons of various training and eating programs and come to a solid science-based decision on how to manage your particular health needs and goals. This course emphasizes the need to understand the science that underlies these lessons. This course will help you understand that our bodies require different food and beverage intake in order to perform our best, maximize our use of calories, and recover the healthiest ways possible. ■

Fueling Up for Fitness Routines
Lecture 1

These 6 lectures on health and fitness will provide you with some tools to examine the pros and cons of various training and eating programs and will help you come to science-based decisions on how to manage your particular health needs and goals.

Myth: Healthy diets and lifelong exercise guarantee that we can live long and healthy lives.

Nothing can guarantee a long and healthy life, but when it comes to increasing our odds of attaining this desirable goal, nothing beats the combination of a well-balanced diet of fresh, whole foods and lifelong vigorous body movement.

Myth: There is a single healthy way to eat and to exercise that will work for everyone.

You've probably noticed that you eat differently depending on the season of the year, whether you have an illness, whether you are pregnant, and many more variables. When it comes to determining how to fuel up for fitness, follow these 2 general principles: (1) listen to your body, and (2) beware of unscientific fitness fads and anecdotes.

Myth: The best diet for all of us is the 3 square meals a day we traditionally eat in America.

Scientific studies have found that eating multiple smaller meals during the day, instead of fewer larger meals, results in less unwanted weight gain and a smoother transition of energy output and energy use during exercise.

Myth: It's important to fuel up just prior to exertions so that you will have maximum energy available.

When there is food in the stomach, a very high percentage of your total **cardiac output** is diverted to the stomach and the intestines to aid in digestion. Ideally, you want to take on food to satisfy your needs far enough ahead of your activity so that your stomach is empty by the time you begin your exercise.

Your **pre-workout meal** should be balanced and low in fat, moderate in **protein**, and highest in **complex carbohydrates**. Your total **calorie** intake before and during the activity will vary depending on your size and the intensity and duration of the activity. A general rule of thumb is that a pre-workout snack should be somewhere around 200 calories. If your activity will last longer than an hour, you will need some more light calories during the activity, in particular, a combination of solids and liquids. Keep the quantities well below the **satiety level** so that your stomach can process the food and empty promptly. Aim for about 50 calories totally from carbohydrates for each hour you are exercising and be sure to stay hydrated.

When you are ready to eat a full meal after your workout, a simple guideline to follow is the **healthy plate rule**. Make sure that half or more of your plate is filled with vegetables and fruit; a quarter or less with lean protein,

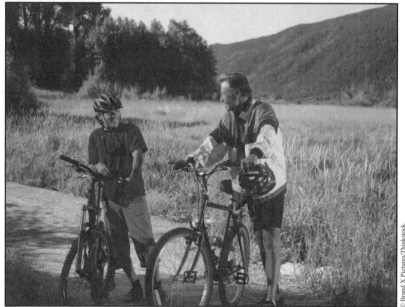

Almost any way you choose to move your body will benefit you. Durations and intensity are secondary to consistency. It doesn't matter if it's skating or rock climbing; running or walking; swimming or snowshoeing; weeding your garden or biking, just make sure it's fun and frequent.

such as fish, poultry, beans, nuts, tofu, or lean cheeses; and the rest, complex carbohydrates, such as grains or whole wheat bread. ∎

calorie: a unit of measure that estimates how much energy is metabolized.

complex carbohydrate: groups of carbohydrates known as polysaccharides; they take longer to be broken down into their component parts than simple carbohydrates do and therefore are a healthier choice.

cardiac output: the volume of blood pumped on each beat of the heart.

Lessons from the Lecture

(1) There is no single diet and exercise program that will work for everyone.

(2) Learn to listen to your body; those signals help find the nutrition and fitness regimen that is optimal for you.

(3) Be skeptical of diet and fitness claims that are not supported by independent, peer-reviewed, double-blind scientific studies.

(4) About 1–2 hours before exercising, eat a light meal of about 200 calories that is low in fat, moderate in proteins, and highest in complex carbohydrates.

(5) During activities that last more than 1 hour, consume an additional 50 calories from carbohydrates for each hour of exercise.

(6) When you're ready to eat after a workout, remember moderation and the healthy plate rule.

Lecture 1: Fueling Up for Fitness Routines

fats: also known as lipids; the most energy dense of all the macronutrients, at 9 calories a gram. They are made up of carbon, hydrogen, and oxygen and function as an energy source, thermal insulator, hunger depressor, and vitamin carrier.

healthy plate rule: a guideline to follow for healthier eating consisting of a plate that is half or more full with vegetables and fruit; a quarter or less with some lean meat such as fish, poultry, beans, nuts, tofu, or lean cheeses; and the rest complex carbohydrates such as grains or whole wheat bread.

pre-workout meal: a light meal 1–2 hours before exercise consisting of about 200 calories, which is low in fat, moderate in proteins, and highest in complex carbohydrates.

protein: from the Greek word *proteios*, meaning "primary." Protein can be found in every tissue in the body; its main function is to build and repair tissue.

satiety level : the amount of food intake that will make you feel full.

Suggested Reading

Benardot, "Timing of Energy and Fluid Intake: New Concepts for Weight Control and Hydration."

Bittman, *Food Matters: A Guide to Conscious Eating with More than 75 Recipes.*

————, *How to Cook Everything: 2,000 Simple Recipes for Great Food.*

Mateljan. *The World's Healthiest Foods.*

"Nutrition and Athletic Performance."

Pollan, *In Defense of Food: An Eater's Manifesto.*

1. What proportions of macronutrients (carbohydrates, proteins, and fats) should make up your pre-workout or pre-race diet in the 4 hours prior to beginning the exertion?

2. Explain why a balanced meal of macronutrients is superior to selecting one or another as the sole source of energy.

Fueling Up for Fitness Routines
Lecture 1—Transcript

Welcome. My name is Dr. Anthony Goodman, and this is the 1st of 6 lectures in our series addressing some of the myths and the realities about the relationship between nutrition and fitness. In these lectures I'll provide you with some of the tools you'll need to examine the pros and cons of various fitness and nutrition programs so you can come to solid science-based decisions on how to manage your particular health needs and goals.

One of the reasons I've been so excited about having this opportunity to present this course is that aside from being a doctor and doing extensive research on scientific aspects of the physiology and the biology of both fitness and nutrition, I've also been involved in sports and competitive activities for virtually my whole life: from the time I played stickball in the streets of Brooklyn as a young boy, to winning international rowing competitions in college, to now, when I am happy to say that my son and his girlfriend taught me to surf for the first time right after my 71st birthday. Being physically fit has mattered, and it still does. In my years of exercise and athletics, I've seen a lot of food and fitness fads come and go. I've also seen plenty of myths around food and fitness take root in popular culture, especially as promoted by celebrities, some medical professionals, and others.

In these lectures on the myths of nutrition and fitness, I think we should begin with perhaps the biggest myth of them all: the great big whopper that says healthy diets and lifelong exercise guarantee that we can live long and healthy lives. I certainly don't want to speak against the value of a healthy diet and of lifelong exercise. I'm all for it for myself, as well as for you. But it's important to know that there is no universal truth here. For example, there are many famous people who lived what we would consider unhealthy lives and thrived at the same time. Winston Churchill comes to mind immediately—he smoked; he drank alcohol; he seemed to be quite sedentary; and he was obese by any measurements. Yet he lived a long, healthy, and mentally active life and he died at the ripe old age of 90.

We have to face the facts that in our quest for health and longevity there are factors beyond our control—for example such things as genetic predispositions. But even if nothing can guarantee a long and healthy life, when it comes to increasing our odds for attaining longevity, nothing beats the combination of a well-balanced diet of fresh whole foods together with lifelong vigorous body movement. There are hundreds of healthy combinations of whole foods, and countless ways to move your body that will all pay enormous benefits.

What I want to do throughout this series is to look at some of the science behind the relationships between dietary choices and athletics, exercise, sports, and just overall fitness. Together we'll take a look at some of the common myths relating to fitness to function, we'll fact-check those myths, we'll examine good science to help unravel the mysteries surrounding those myths, and we'll take a look at what we can learn and apply it in a practical way that can help us all lead healthier lives. Today we're going to talk about fuel for fitness—that is, what foods we should eat to fuel our fitness programs—and also look at when to eat and in what quantities.

But before I offer some specific answers to these questions, I want to stress one very important general theme of all these lectures: We all need to learn to listen to our own bodies. We need to pay attention to the signals that you get from your body; you'll be better prepared if you do this to create ways of eating and moving that work for you, and ways you can modify as you and your circumstances change over time (which they will).

To illustrate this, I want to tell you a true story about something very rare these days: a really cheap flight. This flight goes from New Orleans across the Gulf of Mexico to the Yucatan Peninsula, and takes about 20 hours to fly roughly 500 miles. The flight is cheap because no meals are served en route. This is the annual migratory flight of the ruby-throated hummingbird. This little bird migrates every fall from the American northeast coast to the Yucatan. Normally, this little bird weighs about 5 grams—less than a nickel. It's almost all fluff and feathers. So in the fall it flies south, and then it stops when it gets to New Orleans. It rests there for a couple of weeks and eats like crazy—more than doubling its weight to about 11 grams. Then it takes off to fly non-stop across the Gulf of Mexico. When it arrives in the Yucatan 18 or 20 hours later, it weighs about 6 grams—1 or 2 more grams than its normal weight. This bird has evolved instincts and inner signals which enable it to take on enough fuel for a non-stop flight, plus—as our own 747 jet pilots do—adding enough back-up reserve fuel for head winds and emergencies. It's an astounding piece of nature and it's a miracle of evolution.

My point is that there is a lot that science can teach us about fuel and fitness programs, but we must never forget the importance of listening to our own bodies. Like the ruby-throated hummingbird, our bodies have evolved over millions of years to be responsive to the needs related to survival and optimal performance. Humans needed to be able to run fast and long and hard to either outrun predators or to run down prey. They needed strong muscles for fighting and for defense. Very few animals are as versatile as we are: We can sprint and we can run long distances; we can swim in the water as well as move across the earth at great speeds. Most animals are good mainly in one environment, and we should learn to enjoy and savor that versatility. At the same time avoid abusing our bodies with excesses in diet or exercise.

Let's consider another myth: There is a single healthy way to eat and to exercise that will work for everyone. That is just not reasonable. You will probably have to try more than one way of eating and fitness programs before you settle on the right one for you; and that will also be very likely to change as the years pass, as you and your body change together. Notice that we also tend to eat differently and more depending upon the season of the year—whether we have an illness, whether we're pregnant, and many other variables. Our needs need to and can vary widely, and deserve to be respected.

I'm going to do my best to rely on science whenever possible on defining the best program for you, but there's a lot in this field of nutrition and fitness that changes every single day. What I tell you today and what you choose to adopt today will change over time—sometimes in as little as a few weeks. But listening carefully to the inner guidance from your own body is very useful, and it's the one indicator that you can consistently rely on—especially as scientific studies come and go. So, what does inner guidance look like when we are sitting in front of a bag of our favorite chips, or in my case a box of chocolate-covered raisins? Honestly, it's about learning to know our own limits and our own tolerance, and where you consider yourself to be moderate. It's taking responsibility for feeling good, knowing where you're making good choices and choices for you.

First, let me share a study done on small mammals that clarifies for me what we humans can achieve in learning to listen to our bodies. Many decades ago, biologists studied the diet of a number of different lab animals by giving them a choice of combinations of liquids and nutrients. In each experiment, the animals could choose from identical feeding dishes a diet which would vary in content, calories, and nutrients, but not in taste. The astounding finding was that in almost every case, the animals—lab rats, mice, guinea pigs, and so on—always tended to choose the food dish that had the optimal combination of nutrients for them at that time.

Curt Richter and other pioneering biologists way back in the 1930s showed that even single-celled organisms with no nervous system at all could find their way to the right diet for them. Even slime molds can act in concert with other cells of their own kind to find food; it's absolutely amazing. There are many more of these experiments and observations that support our understanding of animals, ranging from single-celled organisms (like the slime molds) right up to humans, who can self-select the best ways of eating given their own needs for exertion.

However, humans, unlike anything we can study in mice, can also be driven by food cravings. But who's to say that those cravings for that person in that moment? So listening to your own body signals—whether it's about diet or it's about exercise itself—is really the key. Also, with mindful attention after eating and after exercising we can see whether we feel energized or depleted. Did that food give me energy, or did I want to curl up in a ball and go to sleep? Am I really hungry now or am I eating to alleviate boredom, to fill time, or to satisfy an emotional need? In time of emotional stress, we often revert to treats from our childhood days that made us feel warm and safe. The treats our mothers and our fathers gave us when we were sad, or sick. Those are the times to become mindful, to focus on what's really driving your hunger, and even to give ourselves permission to indulge in these comfort foods occasionally, just from time to time.

What I want to offer you are basic scientific principles which should apply across many ages and lifestyles. The challenge is for anyone seriously interested in maintaining good health, good nutrition, and good sports performance, is to stay on top of the current science, and at the same time to avoid like the plague non-tested, popular, nonscientific fads. It's important to be especially alert and skeptical when you see ads or pseudoscientific advice from someone who is trying to sell you something. They may have something of value, but I always suggest that you verify it with independent, peer-reviewed, double-blind prospective studies. Peer review means edited by experts in that particular field of research. Double-blind basically means that the interpreters of the results of the study do not know, for example, who received the actual drug and who received the placebo. Nothing less should satisfy you. When you see an article on muscle-building supplements in a magazine that gets thousands of dollars in advertising from the companies that sell you these supplements, be very careful. So when it comes to determining how to fuel up for fitness, we've already set down 2 general principles: First listen to your body; and beware of those unscientific fitness fads and anecdotes.

Let's turn to some of the specific questions that come up when you are considering how to improve your health and your fitness performance. There are questions to consider about the myths and truths very basic to the whole concept about the kind of fuel and the timing of taking on the fuel before you exercise: what kind of food, how much, and when. First, as to what foods are best for certain sports, it is not clear from current scientific research that there are really significant differences. By and large, if you stick to a fundamentally healthy varied diet, rich in fruits and vegetables, and balanced with complex carbohydrates and proteins, your body will do the adjusting for optimal performance and for better health. I'll get into some of the specifics—such as carbohydrate loading—in another lecture when we talk about some of the extreme forms of exertion and duration. But for most sports, a healthy balanced diet is all you need to consider. This is not difficult; it's not hard stuff.

Let's look at another myth: The best diet for all of us is the traditional American diet of 3 square meals a day. Actually, it is not. Scientific studies have found that eating multiple smaller meals during the day instead of fewer larger meals results in less unwanted weight gain, and a smoother transition of energy output and energy use during the exercise. When we eat this way, we experience fewer valleys and peaks between meals in our blood glucose, and fewer episodes of hunger to drive us to overeating.

Here's another myth: It's important to fuel up just prior to exertion so you will have maximum energy available. In terms of the timing of your meal prior to exercise, the most important factor to keep in mind is that when there is food in the stomach, your body will be focused on the stomach. A very high percentage of your total cardiac output—the volume of blood pumped on each beat of the heart—is diverted to the stomach and to the intestines to aid in digestion, and in the muscular effort required by the stomach and the intestines to grind up your food and move it through more than 40 feet of intestines. This is why after a large meal we often feel listless and sleepy. The digestive processes and the digestive organs are taking priority. This and the rest and restoration phase of your life is taking over. It's not where you want to be when you are getting ready to be vigorous and active. So ideally you want to take on your food or your fuel load to satisfy your needs for that particular effort, but far enough ahead of your activity so that your stomach itself is empty by the time you begin exercise. (When I say stomach, I mean the organ, as opposed to the rest of the intestines which take much longer to empty, but require less energy than the stomach does itself.)

Let's look at the situation when we're considering eating a moderate meal somewhere between 1–2 hours before exertion. Let me qualify that by saying it makes a major difference as to what kind of food you're putting in to your stomach in the first place. For example, if the food is high in fat, it's going to take much longer for your stomach to break down that fat and to get it moving along its way to the intestines where it can be absorbed into the system. That's one extreme. At the other end would be a highly liquid diet such as very watery foods, for example fruits and juices. Those are more rapidly absorbed, along with the sugars or the carbohydrates that they supply to you. Ideally, it's best for your pre-exertion meal to be balanced. By balanced, I mean the meal should be low in fat, moderate in protein, and highest in complex carbohydrates. I'm going to say that several times before our lecture series is over. Why? Because you won't be calling on the fats for energy in the short term, and the protein that you use for rebuilding muscle and other functions can wait until after you have exerted yourself. The carbohydrates are going to be converted into simple sugars which will be used for energy right away, so the carbs should be the highest in the total package in your pre-workout meal for a regular workout routine. (Again, we'll talk about carbohydrate loading for really extreme activities such as marathon running or triathlons in a separate lecture.)

Many coaches and dieticians mention peanut butter sandwiches as a simple, well-balanced meal. They have little fat, moderate protein, and carbohydrates all wrapped in package of complex carbs (ideally in whole grain bread). In fact, some scientists say that if they had to be shipwrecked with only a single food, they would choose peanut butter. It's full of balanced nutrients and relatively nonperishable. However, since peanuts are commonly an antigen to some people, causing allergic reactions, other foods that combine complex carbohydrates with healthy fats and protein are another great option. Some of these include: avocados or hard cheese on a whole grain cracker, eggs with whole wheat toast, turkey and other low fat meats, hummus or other nut butters, all of which add to the variety of choices. Other easy to digest food include yogurt, nuts, fat free milk, and dried fruit. You'll be the final judge of what works for you without that feeling as if you're overdoing your digestive system and making you feel logy.

Finding the balance is what matters, and finding the moderation as well. Eating an unbalanced amount of, for example, protein with the idea that "if a little is good, a lot is better," can have serious and harmful effects. I'll talk more about that a little later. Meanwhile, strive for balance and moderation. A great deal of research suggests that the same rules for your overall nutrition in general will apply to your pre- and post-exercise nutrition as well. A diet high in complex carbohydrates, moderate in protein, and low in fat is, in the long term, the best choice.

Also, take your caloric intake in total before and during the activity. This will be very variable depending upon your size and the intensity and duration of the activity. But a general rule of thumb is that the pre-activity load for a pre-workout snack should be somewhere in the neighborhood of 200 calories. This should be sufficient to prime your energy pump and not bog down your digestive processes. Some examples for that would be a 4 ounce container of low fat yogurt, which has about 115 calories, of which 85 come from sugar; or a small handful of salted peanuts (about an ounce), and that has about 160 calories with very little sugar, and about 7 grams of protein. There are lots of combinations of other choices and other kinds of foods you can put into the mix.

Remember also that your brain needs at least 20 minutes to respond to the signals it gets from a stretched or dilated stomach; so it's easy to overeat if you rush. It is particularly important that you take the time to eat very slowly so your brain can remind you when you've eaten enough—listening to your body. Then you can make use of both the physical signs of stretching of the stomach as well as some of the chemical signals that you'll be receiving without even knowing it. If you want a simple gauge as to the actual volume of food you want to take into your stomach before exercise, just see if the meal or the snack volume is somewhere around the size of your fist. Anything more than that is likely to take too long to move through, and leave you bloated or logy.

Remember, we are all different, and this guide has a wide range of variation depending on your body type, your goals, your levels of exertion, and your endurance. We can unfortunately train our bodies to misbehave. If you habitually overeat—in terms of volume and calories—you will have a chronically overstretched stomach that will not give you the signals of satiety (of fullness) early enough. You will have to re-train by starting to eat multiple small meals during the day to reset the signals to a more healthy level.

It's also probably a mistake to omit all foods prior to exertion. The trick is finding the right fit between too little and too much fuel. For example, if you are an early morning exerciser, then consider a small snack, saving your larger meal for later. We'll talk about that in another lecture about some of the studies on athletes as to timing of food intake. You can do your own experiments, paying attention to the size of a particular meal or snack. (Remember that fist-sized volume of about 200 calories.) Then keep track of how long it takes for the feeling of fullness to disappear. How long is it before you feel that lightness in your body return to you, and you are ready to rumble?

Eating a piece of fruit and/or a piece of toast in the morning, along with a little cheese maybe 30–60 minutes before working out is a good place to start. Feeling yucky? Then the next day, ditch the cheese or the fruit. Does a small bowl of cereal sit better in your stomach? Maybe just a banana? Just experiment. There is no single right way for everyone and every time. I know several high-performance athletes who think the perfect early snack is half a whole wheat bagel (for complex carbohydrates) and a little low fat cream cheese (some protein and a little more fat) topped with a serving of lox (14 grams of protein, almost no fat). Experiment with a small amount of foods that combine fat, carbs, and protein in a healthy ratio. Again, very little fat, more protein, mostly complex carbohydrates.

For me, I know that if I plan a very strenuous exercise session with for example high intensity interval training, along with a weights workout, eating an hour before the workout is really not enough time for me. I feel sluggish at one hour. At 90 minutes I feel substantially better, and in my personal case, 2 hours is my optimal time after a light to moderate midday meal (more than a snack but not quite a "square meal"). For other athletes it's different. You make that judgment by yourself. Perhaps you'd find it helpful to keep a written diet log so you can get a better picture of what works for you. Keeping a log helps because most people can't remember accurately what they've eaten on a specific day.

If your activity will last longer than an hour, say a 2–3 hour bike ride or an all-day, hard, up-and-downhill hike, then you will need even more light calories during the activity. If you are working hard for the entire period of time, staying hydrated as well as stoked with additional sugar is what you'll need. Aim for about 50 or so calories for each hour you are exercising, totally from carbohydrates. This could be, for example, in an easily absorbed form of some kind of healthy sports drink, honey, or just plain sugar. But avoid highly sugared and carbonated drinks.

I'll speak to the issues around maintaining hydration later in a separate lecture, but not to the question of what to eat after your activity—a question which is a little less settled. For routine exercise it may not make any difference what you eat at all. For most of us, the body often signals that it really doesn't want anything—in other words many people find they are just not hungry during the hour or so cool down after a hard or even moderate workout. If you're hungry, go ahead and eat, but eat moderately. You'll never go too far wrong by being alert to those internal signals of real hunger and then responding with moderation. Eat until you are no longer hungry, rather than until you're feeling overly full. Children do this very well; we don't usually do that very well.

When you are ready to sit down to a full meal after your workout, here is another simple guideline that is called by some the healthy plate rule. This healthy plate rule has now replaced the traditional food pyramid. I'm sure this will someday be changed again, but it's an easy-to-follow guide. Make sure your plate—whatever the size of the portion—is filled with at least: 50% or more of vegetables and fruit; about 25% with a healthy source of protein, such as lean meat, fish, poultry, beans, nuts, tofu, or lean cheeses; and about 25% of complex carbohydrates, such a grains and whole wheat bread. Some experts add a little side dish for an extra dose of dairy so that there's a source of calcium in the menu. Remember that this is a different proportion than your pre-workout meal. Take some time to notice the differences in how your body responds to the variety.

A final word on fitness and weight: I am frequently asked if it is better to be overweight and fit than thin and unfit. In my opinion—and the emphasis is opinion—there is no doubt that fitness rises to the top of the list for good health in every way. Being somewhat overweight and vigorously active is way better than being a thin couch potato.

Before we finish, a few things to keep in mind: (1) There is no single diet and fitness program that will work for everyone. (2) Listen to your body; those signals will help you find the nutrition and fitness regimen that is optimal for you. (3) Be skeptical of diet and fitness claims that are not supported by independent, peer-reviewed, double-blind scientific studies. (4) At 1–2 hours before exercising, eat a light meal (fist-sized and about 200 calories) that is low in fat, moderate in proteins, and highest in complex carbohydrates. (5) During activities that last more than an hour, consume an additional 50 calories from carbohydrates for each hour that you're exercising. (6) When you're ready to eat after a workout, remember moderation and the healthy plate rule. Stick with those proportions for fat, protein, and carbs.

Almost any way you choose to move your body will benefit you. Duration and intensity are secondary to consistency. If it's skating or rock climbing, running or walking, swimming or snowshoeing, weeding your garden or tennis—just make sure it's fun and frequent. And as to nutrition, there is no need to have a separate program for daily meals and another for training. Both should be balanced and filled with healthy delicious fresh whole foods. Only the timing and the proportions and the portion size will differ. So go out there, eat well, and make sure to have fun.

Thank you.

Hydration for an Active Life
Lecture 2

This lecture reviews how we should manage our consumption of water and electrolytes, which are the dissolved molecules that we need in addition to the water itself.

Myth: Thirst is a poor indication of dehydration.

Thirst signals any imbalances of the osmolality of our fluids and tissues, which is the concentration of important electrolytes, especially sodium. It is certainly not a late signal of dehydration, coming only after the body has entered the danger zone.

Water makes up about 60–65% of the total body mass in a normal human adult. It is stored in 3 important spaces: (1) the **intravascular space**, which is all the blood cells and plasma inside the blood vessels; (2) the **interstitial space,** which is the space between the cells, and (3) the **intracellular space**, which is the space inside the cells.

Our tolerance for losses or increases in fluids and electrolytes can make the difference between excellent cellular performance, poor cellular performance, cell death, and in extreme cases,

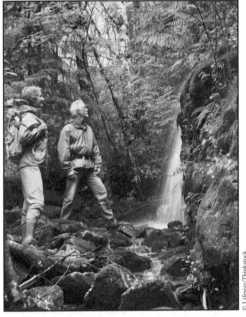

© Lifesize/Thinkstock.

If you are out in nature, bring water with you. Don't drink water found in mountain streams or creeks. There is virtually no place left on Earth where you can assume untreated water is safe. That clear cold stream can be brimming with clear cold parasites and clear cold bacteria.

death of the whole organism. The body is in a constant state of **dynamic equilibrium**, in which fluids are shifting back and forth for redistribution to where they are needed. And the body maintains a strict limit on how much it will allow us to change these volumes and concentrations to prevent serious loss of function.

The body desperately tries to maintain the exact volume in all 3 of the interior spaces. It is crucial to find ways to support that effort when our activities cause even minor shifts. The body will compensate, but it won't be at its most efficient until it's back in balance.

Before starting an activity, avoid having a lot of water inside your stomach; start drinking water a couple of hours before the activity so that you are able to spread out the absorption and fill all your body spaces to capacity.

The body always wants to return to that balanced **internal milieu**. For normal athletic events and outings in moderate temperatures and altitudes, it should be enough to hydrate slowly over several hours and be able to perform well without further input.

Myth: Athletes should avoid caffeine, because it is a diuretic.
Caffeine is a very weak **diuretic**, but there are better ways to hydrate than with a caffeine-containing drink. If you do drink something containing caffeine, you will probably get more fluid from the drink than you will lose from the caffeine.

Myth: Bottled water is the purest, safest, best-tasting source of water.
Bottled water is not necessarily purer, safer, or better tasting than tap water in most cities throughout the industrialized world. If the taste of your local water bothers you, try a carbon filter or reverse-osmosis filter on your faucet. ■

Important Terms

diuretic: something that stimulates increased urine output.

dynamic equilibrium: where fluids are shifting back and forth for redistribution to where they are needed at any specific time and for maximum efficiency.

Guidelines for Rehydration

Rough guidelines for rehydration before, during, and after exercise are outlined below. Remember that you will need to individualize these guidelines by careful trial and error, measuring your intake, urine output, weight, and time periods of activity.

Break your water fast when you wake up in the morning. You don't want to start the day dehydrated.

In the 2–3 hours before you begin your exercise or competition, drink about a quart and a half of water or sports drink. It takes about an hour for a quart and a half of water to leave the stomach and find its way to tissues, especially to muscle.

During your exercise period, aim for about 10–15 ounces every 15–20 minutes for the duration of a long, hard workout.

If the exertion is longer than an hour, you may need to add something more than water, including a drink with about 10% carbohydrates—simple sugars are best—and sodium at about .5 to .7 g/L.

After exercise, you should measure your weight loss and replace it by 150%. By weighing yourself, you will be measuring all the water lost though metabolism, sweat, and obligatory urine loss. If you lose a pound of weight (almost all water) you need to replace it with 1.5 pounds of water or 24 ounces. As a backup, weigh yourself again after you think you have replaced all the water loss, and correct any discrepancies.

internal milieu: term to describe the internal environment of cells.

interstitial space: the space between the cells. It holds about 10–12 quarts of water.

intracellular space: the water and salt inside your cells. This makes up about 25 quarts, a very large percent of the body's total water. Very critical in the management of cell function.

intravascular space: both blood cells and plasma inside our blood vessels, the most critical place for circulation, respiration and oxygenation, delivery of energy containing compounds, and the removal of wastes.

Lessons from the Lecture

(1) Thirst is a good, if not perfect, indicator of dehydration.

(2) Our bodies have a very limited ability to adapt to changes in water content and distribution in and around our cells. So we need to stay very much on top of this issue.

(3) Your job as an athlete is to make sure your body has just a little more fluid and salt than it needs to compensate for the losses you will incur during exercise.

(4) How much and when to drink before and during exercise depends on the duration of the activity, the amount of exertion involved, and environmental conditions like temperature and humidity.

(5) After exercising, measure weight loss and drink enough water to replace 1.5 times the pounds lost.

(6) Tap water is generally as pure and safe as bottled water, and it is certainly safer than water from a stream or other untreated source.

Stover and Murray. "Drink Up!: The Science of Hydration."

Questions to Consider

1. How does the human body store excess water for emergency use compared with the camel? How does this affect pre-exertion fluid planning?

2. Discuss the differences between intravascular fluid, intracellular fluid, and intercellular fluid. How do these spaces contribute to stabilization of the internal milieu?

Hydration for an Active Life
Lecture 2—Transcript

Welcome back. Today we're going to talk about the issues around how we can manage our consumption of water, as well as the salt and electrolytes which are the dissolved molecules that we need in addition to the water itself.

There is a long history of changing ideas about hydration. This is a great example of how important it is to not get stuck with old ideas. When things change for the better and are based on sound scientifically proven principles, we need to be ready and able to make changes. Let me give you an example of how training methods regarding hydration changed in a relatively few decades. Back in the 1950s and 1960s, it was standard practice to not allow competing athletes in many high-exertion and long-endurance sports to drink any water shortly before or especially during the competition. The rationale was that water might cause nausea and stomach cramps and do more harm than good, and that it wasn't necessary anyway.

Fifty years ago, my college experience rowing in 8-oared crew races involved a maximum exertion and energy expenditure for relatively long periods of time. And at no time did we ever have water to drink in the boat. The result was that on one occasion, in 94° heat, between the start of the semifinals race and the finish of the finals 4 hours later, I lost 14 pounds; that's 7 quarts of water and salt! But in competition in those days, everybody was doing the same thing; so that kind of super-dehydration tended to even out in everyone's performance.

Clearly this was not good physiology, but it took a long time for the penny to drop and for old habits to be replaced by new ideas and new information. Over the next several decades the importance of adequate hydration became very apparent. Coaches let go of the old ideas about possible dangers of stomach cramps, and moved on to recognize the benefits of hydration before competition and continuous hydration during competition whenever possible, such as in a marathon. Let's move on now to learn a bit more about how hydration and dehydration works physiologically. Then we can understand how to manage our fluid intake so we can optimize our physical and mental performance.

Let's look at our first myth: Camels survive long periods of dehydration and hot environments by storing water in their humps. No, actually, they don't; and neither can you. The truth is camels store fat in their humps for use when the food is scarce. Their water is stored in other sites such as their tissues and cells. Additionally, they have evolved other protective measures—which we have not—measures designed to improve survival in a severely dehydrating environment. For example, they have oval-shaped red blood cells adapted to move their blood through their vessels even when the blood becomes more thick or viscous from lack of water. And camels can stand a great deal more dilution than we can when they store excess water in their body fluids. This excess in human beings would cause very dangerous dilution changes in osmolality (which is the concentration of dissolved molecules in the fluids). These might cause our cells to rupture, or at least become dysfunctional metabolically. So when the camel stores a lot of water, he can use it later on when he becomes relatively dehydrated. We can't; we are too sensitive to changes in osmotic pressure and fluid volume. Enough about camels.

Here is the mythical whopper of the day: Thirst is a poor indication of dehydration. Sports trainers and many sports journals widely promote the idea that the signal of thirst occurs after you are already significantly dehydrated. So, they are saying, that if you are thirsty, you are already way behind in fluids. This is a very hard thing to quantitate and to study in a scientific way because there are many definitions of the degree of dehydration, as well as when an individual is thirsty. It is also hard to study what is adequate hydration in any individual, as peoples' tolerances vary. Very hard to quantitate data scientifically, so I'll give you my professional opinion (emphasis on opinion). It just doesn't make sense to me and to others that the strongest signal for a possibly life-threatening condition, and at the very least, a performance-threatening condition, should come late among our physiological danger signals. And in our case, thirst is our only readily apparent signal.

Of the many ways we can measure or become aware of dehydration, thirst is the only one that every animal can perceive without any other sophisticated measurements. Thirst signals any imbalances of—first and most importantly—the osmolality of our fluids and our tissues (which, as I just mentioned, is the electrolyte concentration of important items, such as sodium), and then next, the total amount of water in our body (our volume). Just remember that anything that impairs our ability as a species for flight, fight, or overall survival performance is well maintained in evolution, and very high on the list of survival mechanisms. It goes against all scientific logic that this would be a late signal, coming only after we have entered into the danger zone.

So how do our bodies deal with maintaining optimal hydration? Let's just make a quick review of the physiology of where our water is stored. (If you want more detail, you can find it in my lecture series called *How We Fail and How We Heal*.) In a nutshell, in a normal human adult, water makes up about 60–65% of the total body mass. So water is the single most abundant material in the body—a little over 40 quarts. There are some differences between men and women, and adults and children, but for our discussion, I'll round off the differences since it won't affect how we handle fluid maintenance.

Essentially, there are 3 important spaces where the body stores its water. First, the intravascular space (meaning literally "inside the vessels"). This is all the blood (both blood cells and plasma) that's in our arteries, our veins, and our capillaries—the most critical place for circulation, respiration and oxygenation, delivery of energy containing compounds (like glucose), and the removal of wastes. This whole space totals about 5 quarts. And about 3 of those quarts are basically water and dissolved molecules. The remaining 2 quarts in this space are blood cells, which also contain water. This total intravascular volume is especially critical in the athlete (as it would be needed in fleeing a saber-toothed tiger) because this space comes under the great demands during the performance in every physical activity.

Next, there is the interstitial space which you can picture as between the cells, like mortar between bricks. It holds about 10–12 quarts of water—very variable, but a big number all by itself.

Finally, there is the intracellular space, which is the water and salt inside your cells. This makes up about 25 quarts—a very large percent of the body's total water. Maintaining balance in this space is very critical in the management of cell function and performance. The intracellular space contains not only the little organelles that make the cells function, but a great deal of fluid and other molecules that are involved in the thousands of different jobs our cells perform. The importance of this space for this discussion, is that it is very, very finely tuned, and it requires minute correction of every single molecule inside our cells (unlike the camel).

Fortunately, all we have to do is listen to our bodies and supply the water as is needed, and the autonomic systems will take over without you having to do anything. Our bodies' tolerance for water losses or increases in fluids and electrolytes can make the difference between excellent cellular performance, poor cellular performance, cell death, and in the extreme case, the death of the whole organism (us).

Our bodies don't tolerate much of a change of volume in that intracellular space or its osmolality. The important point here is not the exact numbers in each space, but the fact that the body is in a constant state of what's called dynamic equilibrium. Those fluids are shifting back and forth for redistribution to where they are needed at any specific time, and for maximum efficiency. And over the eons of evolution, the body has become very focused on maintaining a strict limit on how much it will allow us to change those volumes and the concentrations to prevent serious loss of function.

For example, one of the things our body does do for us automatically is to shrink the intravascular compartment itself—the volume inside our blood vessels—so when there's not enough blood and fluid inside the arteries, the veins also can maintain normal blood pressure. For example, if you have dehydration or even outright bleeding, the vascular space has the ability to use the muscles in the vessel walls to contract, and the total vascular space is temporarily smaller. This enables the body to maintain blood pressure and blood flow for some variable period of time. This time will depend on the condition of your vessels, the health of your heart, and the degree to which you are dehydrated, and for how long.

If you are young and strong and well-trained, don't get too false a sense of confidence. Doctors learned bitter lessons in dealing with healthy young men during the First and Second World Wars. When the older bodies or the unhealthy, unfit bodies lose blood and fluid, their systems show immediate signs of distress. Blood pressure falls; pulse rises; and those people may go into shock early, but gradually, and fortunately with lots of warning. But in the young and the healthy and the fit, the body for better or for worse has a very strong backup system. For example, the vascular system of the young soldiers would hold together under tremendous physical demands, whereas in an older person, symptoms indicating shock due to dehydration or blood loss quickly become apparent. So in the World War II situation, the GI who was bleeding severely or who was seriously dehydrated might not show signs of shock—falling blood pressure, rising pulse, and so on—until it's too late. And then the whole system would fall apart with little or no warning (except, perhaps, for a sudden cardiac arrest). Older or less fit people would show those signs early on before collapse. Just a fair warning: In very extreme conditions such as those that occur with any combination of very high levels of exertion, and/or extreme temperatures, and extremely long duration, and/or high altitudes, the young and the healthy might get into serious trouble more unexpectedly than someone older or less fit. More about that in a separate lecture where I'll deal with extreme exertion sports and extreme environments.

The upshot of this little physiology lesson is that our bodies don't really tolerate changes in these compartments very well. Our body desperately tries to maintain the exact volume in our intravascular space (inside our blood vessels), as well as in the spaces inside the cells and between the cells. It is crucial to find ways to support that effort when our activities cause even minor shifts in levels of hydration. The body will compensate, but it won't be at its most efficient until it's back in balance.

So, again, the lesson here is that truly we are not camels. However, we do have a few safety valves that help us get by for short periods of time, but these can reach dangerous levels rather quickly under stress, as I suspect was in the case of my own crew races. And in fact, it was not uncommon in those days for oarsmen to collapse at the end of a particularly long race, such as a 4-mile, 20-minute race. We just thought that was normal. It was crazy.

When I lost 14 pounds of water rowing 2 hard races in one very hot day, I had lost nearly 10% of my body weight. That's about 5 times what is considered safe today. But I was 20 years old and it didn't hurt me. If I did that today, in my 70s, it could lead to life-threatening drop in blood pressure and I might die from it.

On the other hand, my body is still pretty smart, and would probably give unmistakable signals to stop me before I got into danger: such as severe fatigue, muscle weakness, and light-headedness much earlier than when I was racing at 20. It would be up to me to take those signals seriously. At 20 I got away with it for much longer. I even won some gold medals. But at 70, those signals, if they go unheeded, might actually be fatal for me. So the lesson here is that we all need to be vigilant when we are out there pushing our bodies to their limits.

Now to the real question: Once you understand that we have a very limited supply to adapt to changes in our water content and distribution, what's the best way to prepare ourselves for exercise? When should we drink our water? How much? And what if anything should be in that water? Keep reminding yourself, "I am not a camel. I cannot store water. I have very little reserve. I need to be ahead of the curve."

For the ordinary athlete who's preparing for some body movement and exertion, most of us can take enough fluid before the event to hydrate us without any needing any further water during the activity. The body will set in motion techniques to preserve water until you can rehydrate yourself. This involves asking the kidneys to reabsorb more water instead of turning it into urine and getting rid of it. But just for a while. There are other more complicated physiologic changes that the body will use to buy time, such as regulating the retention or excretion of sodium, bicarbonate, and chloride, and also redistributing the molecules to maintain near optimal osmolality or concentration. It's helpful to know that the kidneys function under what's called "obligatory water loss," just as a normal part of its operating. You lose about a quart of water per day just sitting still.

What are the practical implications? What can you do? One of the things we want to avoid is to have a lot of water inside our stomachs. (I'm talking again about the organ, the stomach, not your abdomen.) Almost everybody knows how uncomfortable we feel when we take a big swig of water and then try to do something physical. Our stomachs will rebel, either by making us feel uncomfortable, making us vomit, or in some cases giving us severe cramps. So we would really like to have our stomachs nearly empty of actual water volume by the time we begin our exercise. If we start drinking water a couple of hours before our activity, we will be able to spread out the absorption and fill all our body spaces to capacity. Then, remember that the distribution of water and electrolytes within your system is going to be very, very carefully monitored by all sorts of chemical, osmotic, and physical sensors throughout the body.

The body's first concern will be to maintain what the famous French physiologist, Claude Bernard, called, "the constancy of the internal milieu." Imagine a lake into which a river is flowing, and out of which another river is flowing. If even a drop per minute more water enters the lake than leaves it, the lake will eventually overflow; if a drop more water exits the lake than enters it, then the lake will dry up. The same is true of the body. The body needs absolutely perfectly balanced intake and outflow of all its fluids. Your job as the athlete will be to make sure your body has just a little more fluid and salt than it needs for any given losses that you may incur during your exercise. After that your body will rearrange the differences.

How much is that? I suppose the glib answer is "a little more than you need." The body is not going to let you over do it. Remember, your bodies want to come back to that balanced internal milieu, so when there is any variation from the optimum hydration, volume, and osmolality, the body will immediately use it sensors to determine when you've reached your maximum fluid intake, and it will reward you by suggesting strongly that you urinate any excess water and salts. That's the signal you're looking for: a nice copious volume of dilute, light-colored urine prior to the beginning of your exercise. But filling up on huge amounts of water before an event is not going to work. You're either going to make yourself physically sick, get those stomach cramps, or just waste a lot of time trying to urinate out the excess (and hopefully not during the event).

For normal athletic events and outings in moderate temperatures and altitudes, it should be enough to hydrate slowly over several hours to be able to perform well without further intake. The more difficult challenge really comes with activities when you're going to be losing a lot of water from both the extreme exertion and the internal metabolic fire that you are working up inside your abdomen during your training sessions, along with whatever water you happen to be losing through sweat. I'm now talking about a much higher level of intensity.

Let's focus for a minute on sweating. This is not the body's way of regulating water balance, but rather its way of cooling you and maintaining a normal temperature by evaporation. Don't forget that in very dry climates and high altitudes (which we'll talk about in our lecture on extreme conditions), your body still cools itself by sweating, but the sweat may evaporate so quickly that you never notice it on your skin. You can lose large amounts of water without ever really noticing it. Quite different from the way you would, for example, if you are running in a marathon in the middle of summer in Florida, when you would be drenched in sweat and made very aware of the inefficiency of your cooling mechanism, because your sweat just doesn't evaporate fast enough. The only practical way to keep from getting behind in the extreme sporting event or in extreme weather conditions is to continuously take in water during the course of your exercise, at a rate and in quantities that can be absorbed without causing cramps or discomfort. Again, you will find this amount for yourself by careful trial and error.

Remember that while the stomach is not usually the place where water is absorbed in the normal course of events, it can be the place for absorption under urgent conditions. Normally, we absorb water in the small intestine and the colon. If the body needs water urgently it won't wait until it arrives in the small intestine or the colon to start absorbing the water. It will absorb some water right through the walls of the stomach if the osmotic pressure gradient demands it, as it might in dehydration.

For many sports this isn't a problem. If you're playing basketball, baseball, football, or other team sports where you may spend part of the time sitting on the bench, you can sit down and replenish your fluids a little bit at a time while you're resting. At the other end of the spectrum, consider very long sporting events, such as marathons or a triathlon, which can last several hours and in which there is no time spent resting on the bench. In this situation, athletes usually get drinks of water along the way from kind people or trainers handing them cups of water. I think the more water you can comfortably get right into your system during the event, the better—as long as it isn't so much as to produce cramps or nausea. I'll mention some guidelines about that too, before we're finished here.

For the moment, let's look at another myth: Athletes should avoid caffeine because it's a diuretic (something that stimulates increased urine output), so it might make you lose more water than you are taking in. This is really only partly true. Caffeine is a very weak diuretic; that's why doctors don't use caffeine as a diuretic for the patients who might need one. There are far better ways to hydrate than with a caffeine-containing drink, but if you want to hydrate with a drink containing some caffeine, go ahead. You're probably going to get more fluid from the drink than you will lose from the caffeine. The same is not true of alcohol. Alcohol is very dehydrating and you will get dehydrated much faster.

Here are a few of my rough guidelines for rehydration before, during, and after exercise. For the very serious competitive athlete: You will need to individualize hydration by careful trial and error, and by measuring your intake, urine output, weight, and time periods. For the rest of us: We need to listen to our bodies' needs, our own energy, notice our feelings of thirst, light-headedness, and nausea. These are all important indicators. For all of us: In the 2–3 hours before you begin your exercise or competition, drink about a quart and a half of water or sports drink. Also remember to break your water fast when you wake up in the morning; you don't want to start the day dehydrated. Keep in mind it takes about an hour for a quart and a half of water to leave your stomach and find its way to your tissues, especially to your muscles. During your exercise period, aim for about 10–15 ounces every 15–20 minutes for the duration of the long, hard workout. If the exertion is longer than an hour, you may need to add something more than water, including a drink with about 10% carbohydrates (simple sugars are the best) and sodium at about 0.5 to 0.7g/L. For that you're going to have to read the label. For more information about sports drinks, you'll want to check out the lecture in this series on supplements and fitness.

After exercise you should consider measuring your weight loss and replacing it by 150%. By weighing yourself, you will be measuring all the water lost though metabolism, sweat loss and obligatory water loss. What weight you lose by burning fat is not enough to change the equation, so don't worry about that. If you lose a pound of weight (almost all water), you need to replace it with 24 ounces of water, which is 1.5 pounds of water. Those are rough guidelines for everyone, but ultimately you will want to know and regulate your own personal optimal fluid intake. Everybody sweats at a different rate; this is where you will be responsible for knowing your own body, and keeping track of your tank and keeping it topped off throughout the period of exertion.

So in a word, if you want to fine-tune your fluid intake, I suggest that you weigh yourself naked before you workout, then again naked right afterward (this is to eliminate the error you'll incur if you have half a pound or more of sweat still in your workout clothes). Keep a record of your weight losses and the volume of water it represents; and make sure to note whether this was an average effort or an especially hard one, and how hot it was. You'll see the pattern very quickly and know just how much to replace. Remember to replace it by 1.5 times the amount you have lost. As a backup, weigh yourself again (naked) after you think you have replaced all the water loss, and then correct any discrepancies.

A final word about one source where I do not recommend you get your water. If you are out in the magnificence of nature, perhaps hiking or enjoying a cross-country run, and there is a mountain stream with an abundance of beautiful, cold, clear, running water at your feet, don't even think about drinking it! Pour it over your head; pour it over your clothes if it feels good; get in it and swim in it. But don't drink it! There is, to my great sorrow, virtually no place left on Earth where you can assume untreated water is safe. That clear cold stream can be brimming with clear, cold parasites and clear, cold bacteria. Humans pollute them; animals pollute them; and there's no good way to know if it is safe to drink or not. You need to take your own purification with you, or carry your own water.

For the final myth of this subject: Bottled water is the purest safest best-tasting water in the world. In a nutshell, there is no value in bottled water at all. It's not necessarily purer or better-tasting than tap water. In most cities throughout the industrialized world tap water is perfectly safe and pure. Bottled water costs more than gasoline, and literally thousands of times more than tap water—not to mention the horrific carbon footprint caused by bottling and shipping the water around the world. It is in my opinion, pure nonsense. If the taste of your local water bothers you, get a carbon filter and make your own water taste good. As to other elements and possible contaminants in tap water, this will vary by city and by the filter type. Carbon filters make water taste better, but not much else. Reverse osmosis filters are at the other end of the spectrum and remove almost everything harmful from the water. Of course, in places without reliable water purification, bottled water or some system of purification makes sense.

A few points to highlight as we wrap up. (1) Thirst is a good, if not perfect, indicator of dehydration. (2) Our bodies have a very limited ability to adapt to changes in water content and distribution in and around our cells. (3) Your job as an athlete is to make sure your body has just a little more fluid and salt than it needs to compensate for the losses you will incur during exercise. (4) How much and when to drink before and during exercise depends on the duration of the activity, the amount of exertion involved, and environmental conditions such as temperature, altitude, and humidity. (5) After exercising, measure weight loss and drink enough water to replace 1.5 times the amount of weight you've lost. (6) Tap water is generally as pure and safe as bottled water, and it is certainly safer than water from a stream or other untreated source.

There are some events and times when you may get behind in fluids or sources of energy. It could be in long distance endurance sports, or in just getting stranded in the wilderness, unprepared for injury or a change in the weather. On extended hikes or full days in extreme temperatures, I always carry extra water or a portable water filter for outings of more than a day. And finally, a portable stove for melting snow or purifying water in cold winter conditions can be helpful, too. In the end, most of these situations are preventable or can be fixed by taking responsibility for being prepared ahead of time. I always suggest the test question should be: "Which mistake would I rather make: Being over-prepared and not needing it, or being under-prepared and desperately needing it?" It's your choice. Now you have a wide range of options to keep you safely hydrated while you enjoy your athletic endeavors.

The Skinny on Exercise and Weight Loss
Lecture 3

This lecture focuses on those of us who want to lose a moderate amount of weight, in the range of 10 to 30 pounds, or those who wish to maintain their weight. In the area of severe obesity, weight loss should be guided by a physician and a professional dietician.

Myth: Anyone can lose weight and keep it off.
The bad news is that the recovery rate from **obesity** is abysmally small. But the good news is that if you are strongly motivated and determined, you can lose excess weight without torture or horrible deprivation.

The U.S. National Weight Control Registry found that the key in 98% of successful dieters was making major changes in total food intake. Additionally, 94% increased their physical activity, mostly through simply walking more.

Myth: You can control and improve your weight by either piling up on or entirely eliminating 1 of the 3 macronutrient food groups—fat, protein, or carbohydrates.
Eating properly and controlling weight is all about balance, proportion, and quality. For example, some diets suggest entirely eliminating carbohydrates. Fast-acting carbs, such as white breads, candies, and juices, have a high **glycemic index** and can create weight gain. However, complex, slow-acting carbohydrates, such as vegetables and whole grains, aid digestion and are important sources of fiber and nutrition.

The small grain of truth underlying many of these so-called miracle diets is that it is possible to lose some weight quickly in the first few weeks or months. But that weight loss often comes merely as water loss, particularly in low-carb diets.

Caloric balance is simply a matter of subtraction and addition: If you eat more calories than you burn, you will gain weight; if you burn more than you eat, you will lose weight.

Myth: We just need a little will power in the amount of food we consume, and we can weigh whatever we want to.

Throughout millions of years of evolution, the greatest survival threat to virtually all organisms was and is starvation. Even the slightest decrease in caloric intake or slight loss of weight will be detected by the body, and combated as if our lives depended upon it—because for millions of years, they did! The battle to lose weight and maintain that weight loss revolves around bypassing these strong survival instincts while remaining healthfully lean and strong.

Myth: You can use exercise alone to achieve weight loss.

A pound of energy in your body comes to an average of 3500 calories, or if it's pure fat you want to lose, about 4000 calories. An average adult male weighing 155 pounds, doing 30 minutes of moderate to vigorous exercise 3 times a week would burn 600–800

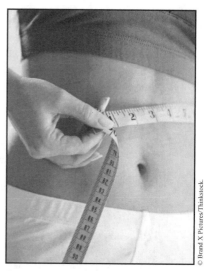

If you are strongly motivated, focused, and determined, you can lose excess weight without torture or horrible deprivation.

calories a week. The number of calories you are able to burn in any given period of exertion is relatively small, and in some people, exercise actually stimulates the appetite in the body's effort to stave off weight loss.

Some studies seem to show a definite correlation between the maintenance of weight loss, rather than the loss of weight, and exercise. Once they get the weight off, people who keep on exercising tend to maintain that weight loss.

Myth: It matters when you choose to eat your calories. One popular idea is that if you eat before going to bed or late at night, you will gain more weight.

Many well-done scientific studies have shown that it makes absolutely no difference in the long run what time of day you take in your calories. One small study, however, has found that it may be better to exercise in a fasting state—before you've eaten any breakfast—if you want to lose recent weight gain and stave off some of the dangerous side effects of overeating.

Myth: It is possible to reduce fat selectively on our bodies.

There is absolutely nothing you can do to remove unwanted fat from specific areas of your body, because fat distribution is encoded in your DNA. The key is to maintain a healthy **body-mass index** and enjoy body movement. Direct your energy and your workouts to maintaining a healthy weight and overall strength, flexibility, and stamina. ■

Lessons from the Lecture

(1) Don't waste time and money on the newest fad diet or the huge number of unscientific exercise myths such as spot reduction.

(2) Losing weight is all about calories eaten and calories burned. To lose weight successfully, you will need to burn more and eat less—and you will need to keep on exercising.

(3) Don't try to time how and when to eat. Timing probably won't get you anywhere.

(4) Stick to the science and not anecdotes.

(5) Don't forget to make use of the professionals out there before making major changes to your diets or your exercise routines.

body-mass index: the gold standard of population-based measurements of overweight. Take your weight in pounds, multiply it by 703, and divide by your height in inches squared; a BMI of less than 24.9 is considered normal weight, between 25 and 29.9 is overweight, and greater than 30 is obese.

glycemic index: a measurement of how quickly blood sugar rises after the ingestion of a particular carbohydrate food.

obesity: any body mass index of greater than 30. The 3 different types of obesity that have been defined are hypercellular, hypertrophic, and hyperplastic.

Suggested Reading

"Calories burned in 30 minutes for people of three different weights."

"Nutrition and Athletic Performance."

Olshansky, Passaro, Hershow, et al. "A Potential Decline in Life Expectancy in the United States in the 21st Century."

Robbins and Ornish. *The Food Revolution.*

Roizen and Oz. *You Staying Young.*

Taubes. *Good Calories, Bad Calories.*

"U.S. Obesity Trends."

Questions to Consider

1. Explain why diets that focus on a single macronutrient are likely to fail. How do these diets compare with overall success rates?

2. What has been the effect of evolution from early primates to current humans with regard to the starvation signals and diet?

The Skinny on Exercise and Weight Loss
Lecture 3—Transcript

Welcome back. Today we're going to look at weight loss and its relationship to fitness and nutrition. I'm going to concentrate on those of us who want to lose a moderate amount of weight, let's say around the range of 10–30 pounds, or those who simply wish to maintain their already healthy weight. I won't get into the area of severe obesity, also known as morbid obesity, because those who want to or need to lose 100 pounds or more should be under the care of a physician and a professional dietitian. The guidelines and safety issues for that kind of weight loss are not the same as in moderate weight loss. For more detailed information specifically on severe obesity, let me refer you to my lectures on lifelong health.

First I want talk about a group of myths around weight loss as opposed to healthy weight maintenance that have grown together in the minds of many people. These are myths perpetuated by anecdotal evidence, which in the world of medical science we like to call "The Big Lie." Remember again, when we are dealing with pseudo science, especially from people who would like to sell us something—a book or a program or a supplement to improve our health—the number of anecdotes or testimonials is totally irrelevant regarding the quality of the product. I'm sure you've all seen or read ads where individuals claimed to have lost tons of weight in a short period of time by taking a certain pill or supplement and then watching the fat melt away. Just remember: A thousand anecdotes is as useless as one anecdote. Anecdotes and testimonials are not scientific data. The commercial diet world is overflowing with them because so many people struggle with maintaining a healthy or cosmetically approved weight.

Let's start at the top of the list of myths: Anyone can lose weight and keep it off. Don't I wish? First, the bad news: Statistics indicate that 95% of people who lose weight in the short term (say over a period of 4–6 months) will be back at their pre-diet weight by the end of the first year. The good news is that if you are strongly motivated, focused, and determined, you can lose the excess weight without feelings of constant deprivation—and you can keep it off. It isn't complicated; you just have to learn to pay attention to your body, to the science, and to the whole way of living and eating rather than to fad diets for quick fixes.

Let's look at some of the data from the United States National Weight Control Registry about what successful people did to keep weight off after they lost it. In the population they studied, the main technique for 98% of successful dieters was to make major changes in total food intake. Additionally, 94% increased their physical activity as well. For most of them, this meant simply walking more. The group trying to lose weight lost an average of 66 pounds and kept it off for more than 5 years. The majority of the people in this group reported eating breakfast every day; weighing themselves regularly at least once a week or more; watching fewer than 10 hours of TV a week; and exercising about an hour a day. Note the moderation and the consistency— not deprivation.

Here's another myth that ties right in: We can control and improve our weight by either piling upon, or entirely eliminating, 1 of the 3 main macronutrient food groups (fats, proteins, or carbohydrates). This is completely wrong, and you'll know it right away because there's no balance, and your body will tell you so. For instance, there are some diets that suggest entirely eliminating carbohydrates as a way to lose weight. The idea comes from the fact that simple, fast acting carbohydrates (such as white breads, candies, and juices) all have a high glycemic index, and they can lead to weight gain. That's true, but the complex, slow-acting carbohydrates (vegetables and whole grains) aid digestion and are important sources of fiber and nutrition. Again, it's all about balance, proportion, and quality.

When you have a moment, just check out one of the mega-book stores or go on-line to any of the giant bookseller's websites, and you'll get a rough idea on the number of books on sale for weight-loss dieters. One site I went to had over 50,000 references, and a large bookstore I visited had more than 300 books on dieting alone! Here's something to think about: If even one of those many books really worked in the long term for the majority of people, we would all be reading that book. We would all be using that diet. But we're not; that tells you something important about all the new fads: Most of those diets are non-scientific nonsense.

Also, there are hundreds of published diets out there which tout loading up on carbs or proteins and ditching fats, for example. There is absolutely no science to back up these fads or other kinds of fad diets as well. At best, some of these diets are harmless, but many are not. Some are very risky. The small grain of truth underlying so many of these so-called "miracle diets" is that it is possible to lose some weight very quickly in the first few weeks or months. But that early weight loss often comes merely as water loss, which occurs most often in the low carbohydrate diets—which, by the way, are very unbalanced and very unhealthy ways of eating, and which you cannot safely sustain over the long run. By going to extremes, you may make yourself both very unhappy and probably very unhealthy as well.

Now let's move away from the myth of unbalancing the macronutrients as a way to lose weight and look at some simple, undeniable science. First, and most important: A calorie is a calorie. It makes no difference what food group that calorie comes from, whether it's from fat, carbohydrate, or protein. They are all the same for whatever the body wants to do with them. Evolution has given our bodies complete discretion on how it will deal with fuel. It breaks down everything into smaller molecules and then reassembles exactly what it needs at the moment. You have no say in what the body does with the calories you feed it. Reducing fat, for example, doesn't mean that the body will selectively lose fat as well. Secondly, permanent stable weight loss and weight gain are not matters of complicated calculus or quadratic equations. You don't need a 400 page diet book with tables and charts. Caloric balance is simply a matter of subtraction and addition. If you eat more calories than you burn, you will gain weight. If you burn more calories than you eat, you will lose weight. Period. That alone could be enough information for the whole lecture.

But let's look a little closer by talking about another myth: We just need a little will-power in the amount of food we consume, and we can weigh whatever we want to. It's not that simple. Throughout millions of years of evolution, the greatest survival threat to virtually all organisms was not death at the hands of a predator (being killed and eaten by a 4-legged predator, for example); it was not flood or by fire or by drought; it was not death by infection, disease, or broken bones, or even tribal wars. Of course, all of these were definitely threats to survival, and evolution selected the mechanisms that would give the organism—you and me, in this case—the best odds to survive and to spread our genes to the next generation. The biggest threat of all over eons of time—and still, sadly, in some parts of the world even today—was and is starvation.

Whether we like it or not, our bodies are armed with powerful genes and internal signals and metabolic mechanisms that kick in as soon as our bodies detect anything that suggests we might be headed for a starvation situation. And that means our bodies' regulatory mechanisms will detect even the slightest decrease in caloric intake or slightest loss of weight, and then it will resist it as if our lives depended upon it, because for millions of years it did. The 2 strongest reactions by the body are first, the sensation of hunger and the consequent very strong drive to eat something, anything to satisfy that hunger. Jonathan Swift, the author who wrote *Gulliver's Travels*, said "He was a bold man that first ate an oyster." Well, that man wasn't just bold, he was hungry. The second mechanism in our bodies' drive to stave off starvation: Our metabolic gears will naturally downshift to burning fewer calories in order to maintain a stable weight. Most of us have experienced the initial weight loss when we reduce calories, then we find that the weight loss tapers off after a week or so. Then if we drop the calories some more we lose a bit more weight, and then that, too, tapers off. It's very frustrating. This is more complicated physiologically, but in simplest terms, our bodies reset the internal thermostat, lowering our metabolism so that our internal energy furnaces burn slower and slower to keep us from losing weight. Or, from a purely physiological perspective, to prevent starvation.

The exact resetting is very variable, but we can foil that mechanism by moving and forcing the body to work harder so that the calories-in and the calories-out equation will help us in the weight-loss department. The challenge to lose weight and maintain that weight loss revolves around how we can bypass those strong survival instincts and still remain healthfully lean and strong. And hopefully joyful as well. I say "joyful" because this can and should be a lifelong work in process, and the element of joy will make it sustainable.

Before I get specific, let's look at the big picture. Let's just forget about the whole concept of "dieting" as it's defined by our society: as a way to lose weight, and as a short-term cure for what is really a lifelong issue. You may have heard me say this before, but it bears repeating. We want to think of the Greek origin of the word *diaita*, meaning a way of living, and in our context, also a way of eating. This very critical concept encompasses our whole relationship with food well beyond calories and nutrition, and focuses on balance and on how and when and with whom we eat. In reality, we just need a healthy framework that we can build on so that we can eat moderately, healthfully, and joyfully for the next 20, or 50, or 75 years, without a continuous feeling of hunger and frustration. Once we build that framework, then we ask ourselves, how does it feel, how does it fit, and how does it go within our overall fitness program?

Which leads me to the next myth: We can use exercise alone to achieve weight loss. So after we devour a delicious bacon cheeseburger and fries, you can go to the gym and work it off. Again, I only wish that were true. Let's look at this one carefully. Let's say we want to lose about a pound a week—not an unreasonable goal to start with. A pound of energy in our body comes from an average of about 3500 calories; if it's pure fat you want to lose, then it's 454 grams (in a pound) × 9 calories per gram of fat which equals roughly 4000 calories. And, of course we would rather burn off the fat. That's 4000 calories to burn a week to lose a pound of fat per week.

Now, how many calories do we burn when we're actively moving our body? This will vary a great deal, but let's just look at the average adult male who weighs about 155 pounds, and does 30 minutes of moderate to vigorous exercise (which happens to be the amount of time most people devote to aerobic exercise in a given workout) generally 3 times a week. The approximate calories burned in 30 minutes of a few common activities are: a brisk walk (4 miles per hour, typical treadmill pace) will burn about 160 calories in that 30 minutes; running 5 miles per hour (an 11 minute mile, which isn't too fast) burns about 335 calories over 30 minutes; a rowing machine (a moderate pace, a light load) burns 260 calories; stationary biking burns 225 calories; tennis burns about 260 calories; swimming burns 223 calories.

Three times a week of these very common activities leads to about 600–900 calories burned per week—not per day, per week. Those extra calories burned will help you lose about a quarter of a pound a week. A half-pound bacon cheeseburger with fries and a milkshake could contain 2000–3500 calories. Exercising the next day won't make a dent.

I'm not trying to deter anyone from exercise. There are so many positive aspects about our overall health and happiness regarding regular exercise that I could use up the next 3 lectures on that alone. Burning up an extra quarter of a pound per week will add up over the long term, but it will not balance out regular eating binges. So, yes, keep at it. Keep moving. There is absolutely no question that exercise is the single most effective way to establish and maintain a long and healthy life—both physically and mentally. Exercise can stave off cognitive mental decline, as well as free us from crippling diseases such as arthritis. Moving your body by itself might be the most important single factor in a healthy lifestyle. Combined with a healthy, moderate way of eating, it will serve you best throughout your lifetime.

If you want to use exercise at this relatively average intensity and frequency, it's not likely to pay the dividends you want with regard to losing weight in the short term. On the other hand, there are very few things that will give you as much bang for the buck as a regular, joyful, sustained episode body movement. More on that in a minute.

For now, just remember that the number of calories you are able to burn in any given period of exertion is relatively small, and in some people can actually stimulate the appetite in our bodies' effort to stave off any further kind of weight loss. So why bother? Can we use exercise to lose weight? And just as important: Can you use exercise to maintain weight loss? What does the science say?

In a huge study run by Harvard, more than 34,000 women were observed over a period 13 years, and their dietary habits and weight loss were measured and tracked. This is a big, long-term study. These women averaged about 54 years old at the beginning of the study, so they were in their mid- to late-60s at the end of the study. Most of the women over that 13 years gained weight on the average of about 6 pounds. But some gained a lot more. However there was a subgroup of women in this study who maintained their body weight over that period of time. Most of the women in this leaner group exercised at a very moderate level every day for about an hour or so. This amounted to not much more than walking at a moderately brisk pace, or other forms of similar moderate exercise. But they had done it for many years and started out with lower body weights.

In another study on women, this one with a very restrictive unsustainable diet—800 calories a day (that's nearly a starvation diet)—these women all lost weight. But those in the group that were also on an exercise program tended not to revert to their pre-diet weight once they went back to a more normal way of eating. Those who did not exercise did regain the weight. Interesting, and unexplained so far, was the fact that the new weight gain in this non-exercising group was distributed mostly around their waists. We know this is a particularly unhealthy place to have extra weight, because it's apparently more metabolically active and associated with a higher incidence of coronary artery heart disease.

With these studies on humans, plus many other studies on laboratory animals, there seems to be a definite correlation and benefit between the maintenance of weight loss through exercise, rather than the loss of weight through exercise alone. Once you get the weight off, no matter how you do it, the most constant theme is that the people who keep on moving tend to maintain that weight loss. The sedentary people don't.

The really good news is that much of this benefit can be achieved with fairly modest but consistent levels of exertion. In fact, one study on humans showed that merely standing up for long periods of time without doing any hard exercise increased the amount of energy expended and contributed to a small but statistically significant weight loss.

Another key point to remember is that muscles burn more calories at rest than fat does; the higher muscle to fat ratio, the easier it is to burn calories, too. How much does it help? It's way to variable from person to person and activity to activity to give you an actual number. Just keep moving and think about including some weight training. The takeaway from this is that we really should not be trying to separate fitness and nutrition when it comes to maintaining or achieving a healthy weight.

Now let's look at another myth regarding not just how much we eat, but when we eat. The myth tells us it matters when you choose to eat your calories. One popular idea is that if you eat before going to bed or late at night you will gain weight. This is definitely a myth. Many well done scientific studies have shown that it makes absolutely no difference in the long run what time of day you take in your calories.

From another perspective, however, there's also a possibility that there is a kernel of truth in this food-timing myth. Having just said that you cannot time your food intake to minimize weigh-gaining, let's look at a study from 2010. I would have until recently been the first one to say that you just can't fool Mother Nature with this timing idea, but in a small, but very well done study, researchers in Belgium seem to be suggesting something else. At least in one very short-term study, it seems that it may be better to exercise in the morning in a fasting state—before any breakfast at all—if you want to lose recent weight gain and stave off some of the dangerous side effects of over-eating.

The researchers took a small number of healthy male athletes ages 18–24 years old, and divided them into 3 groups. All 3 groups ate what the researchers called "hyper-caloric fat-rich diet" for 6 weeks. This included a huge 30% increase to their usual total calories, with 50% of these calories coming from fat. Very, very unhealthy. But, remember that these were young, very well-trained healthy athletes, and this diet was not a normal part of their lives. One group exercised 4 mornings a week at very high intensity for either 60 or 90 minutes at a time after an 8–10 hour fast. This group ate only after exercising. A second group ate before exercising and also drank sports drinks with carbohydrates during exercising. Both groups did the same intensity workout and ate the same total amount of calories during the day, except the fasting group took their calories only after they worked out.

The third group—the control group—had the same diet but did no exercise at all. In this control group of experimental couch potatoes (remember, this was not their normal lifestyle, by the way) gained about 6 pounds in the 6 weeks—no surprise there. They became insulin resistant, and fat tended to accumulate inside and outside their muscle cells. Both of these conditions (insulin resistance and fatty muscles) are very unhealthy in the long term.

The second group of exercisers who did eat before and during the exercise gained about 3 pounds (half as much as the controls); they, too, had some impaired insulin and carbohydrate metabolism and some fatty deposition inside their cells. Only the first group of fasting exercisers maintained a healthy level of glucose metabolism and muscle maintenance with almost no weight gain.

Training after a significant fast (8–10 hours) was much more protective of critical metabolic processes in people with short-term unhealthy nutrition than eating before and during exertion. Remember, that this is a very early kind of research; it is a small study; and it revolves around a very specific kind of bad diet and intense exercise program for a very short period of time. In addition, the protection for the fasting group came through very high intensity training for long periods of time (60–90 minutes), 4 days a week—much more intense than the average person could be expected to do.

So far, there is no data as to how this would work in the general population, and whether lower levels of say, mild aerobic training with moderate ways of eating would produce the same effect under these fasting conditions. Don't take this as a license for binge eating and then binge exercising; both are likely to be unhealthy over time. Also, let's not confuse this with another lecture in which I suggested eating about 200 calories an hour or 2 before exercise; there I was referring to maximizing performance, not efforts to lose weight as I am here.

My personal takeaway would be that if I can exercise in the fasting state, especially on days I was going to do high intensity interval training or at least at the upper end of my intensity range of workouts, I would try to do it before breakfast.

Speaking of how we move our bodies, let's look at our next myth: It's possible to reduce fat selectively in specific areas of our bodies. In a word, there is absolutely nothing you can do to remove unwanted fat from specific areas of your body—period. This is one area where your instincts are probably right. Most people who are paying attention notice that they tend to accumulate extra fat in a specific area of their bodies, and that area is where the fat is the last to go after losing weight, and the first to return when you gain weight. Everybody's heads should be nodding now. This is the very nature of your individuality, and you just have to learn to live with it. That hanging flesh or flab under your upper arms will not go away with triceps exercise. Neither will your abdominal paunch (or mine) go away after you've done 10,000 crunches. Fat distribution is encoded in your DNA. Don't waste your time or emotion on trying to change that, just maintain a healthy body-mass index (weight) and enjoy your body movement. Don't waste another minute or another dollar on rubber suits or focal exercise programs aimed at spot reduction; there is no such thing.

So as we conclude this lecture, let's just take a minute to highlight the important points: First, losing weight is all about calories eaten and calories burned. To lose weight successfully, you will need to burn more and eat less, and you will have to keep on moving your body. Secondly, don't waste your time and money on the newest fad diet and the huge number of unscientific exercise myths such as spot reduction. Third, don't try to time how and when to eat. Timing probably won't get you anywhere. Fourth, stick to the science and not anecdotes. And finally, don't forget to make use of the professionals out there before making major changes to diets or exercise routines.

This is all about a life-long pursuit of health and happiness. It is far easier to develop those healthy ways of eating and moving that will meld together and keep you fit for life than to torture yourself for short term gains. Find a way to move your body that's fun and something you can look forward to. Keep it light. Keep it joyful.

Thank you.

Some Facts about Vitamins and Supplements
Lecture 4

For people who maintain a normal and nutritious intake of whole foods, there's no need to depend on extra vitamins and mineral supplementation. The exception to this rule may apply to a few special groups, such as athletes who are on restrictive, unbalanced diets; pregnant women; children who do not eat a fully balanced diet to meet their needs; and menopausal and postmenopausal women, who may need additional calcium.

Myth: It's natural, so it must be healthy.
Some of the most potent poisons on Earth are natural, including belladonna alkaloids and botulinum toxin. Further, lifesaving, naturally occurring drugs, such as digitalis from purple foxglove and even insulin, can be dangerous or lethal if taken in the wrong dose. The key is dose: the proper amount, at the right time, for the right person.

Myth: Athletes need large amounts of protein to increase muscle mass and strength, often taken in the forms of artificial supplements.
Many sports experts, even some doctors, suggest that high-protein diets and protein supplements are necessary, yet it's hard to find scientific evidence that proves this to be true. In fact, very high protein diets (200–400 grams per day) probably exceed the liver's capacity to eliminate excess urea nitrogen.

To achieve balance, you should look at 2 things: (1) the absolute amount of protein in grams per day, and (2) the absolute maximum recommendations, which are roughly 1 gram per pound per day of the body weight—about 175 grams for a 175-pound person—but no more. An evaluation of protein supplements published by *Consumer Reports* found that most people get sufficient protein in their regular diets.

Myth: Creatine enhances growth-promoting substances, enhances energy production, and increases the synthesis of muscle proteins.
Creatine is a naturally occurring molecule; it's found in human organs, muscles, and body fluids. It chemically combines with phosphate molecules

to form something called phosphocreatine, which is a high-energy phosphate and is active in the anaerobic phase of muscular contraction. Creatine is one of the most widely sold supplements, especially among bodybuilders, but does it work?

Researchers found that increased levels of creatine in the muscle might allow for the buildup of stores of phosphocreatine, which could lead to extra energy

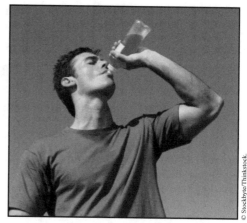

Sports drinks promise better athletic performance, but most are just sugar water.

in the form of **adenosine triphosphate**, or **ATP**. But beyond this theoretical advantage, they were unable to show actual performance improvement. Any benefit at all seems to be limited to very short-duration, high-intensity efforts at the extreme edge of the energy envelope.

Myth: Quercetin is the new miracle substance that will allow us to reach higher performance levels, even without extra training.
Quercetin is a flavonoid compound, one of many found in nature that often have antioxidant and anti-inflammatory properties. It can be found in apple skins, berries, red wine, black tea, and some leafy vegetables. In experiments with mice and quercetin, investigators found some increase in markers of mitochondrial biogenesis, the energy powerhouse in cells. They speculated that this could have implications for human endurance, but human studies show no improvement in performance.

Myth: Sports and energy drinks are a safe and cost-effective way to improve performance and maintain hydration.
Sports drinks are designed to maintain optimal hydration and may also contain carbohydrates and some electrolytes. Energy drinks are similar to sports drinks but also contain stimulants, such as caffeine. You might try

making your own sports drinks with water, fruit juice, some sugar, and salt. As for energy drinks, they likely pose risks associated with caffeine and other stimulants and probably do not improve performance. ■

adenosine triphosphate (**ATP**): molecule found within cells that carries energy.

creatine: a naturally occurring molecule; found in human organs, muscles, and body fluids. It chemically combines with phosphate molecules to form something called phosphocreatine, which is a high-energy phosphate, and is active in the anaerobic phase of muscular contraction.

quercetin: a flavonoid compound, one of many found in nature that often have some antioxidant properties, as well as anti-inflammatory properties. It can be found in apple skins, berries, red wine, black tea, and some leafy vegetables.

Suggested Reading

Arria and O'Brien. "The 'High' Risk of Energy Drinks."

Bilsborough and Mann. "A review of issues of dietary protein intake in humans."

Consumer Reports Ratings. Sports Drinks.

Herbal Research Foundation. "Herbal Stimulants."

Hyman and Liponis. *Ultraprevention*: *The 6-Week Plan that Will Make You Healthy for Life.*

Mayo Clinic. "Caffeine Content for Coffee, Tea, Soda and More."

Mayo Clinic Recommendations for Energy Drinks.

1. What is the value of vitamin supplementation in normal human activities? Preparation for hardcore endurance events?

2. Compare the effectiveness of protein powders, creatine supplements, and quercetin in improving performance in athletics.

Some Facts about Vitamins and Supplements
Lecture 4—Transcript

Welcome back. Today let's go ahead and dive right in to one big myth: Multi-vitamins and supplements are necessary to achieve and maintain optimal health and well-being, and to improve athletic performance. The truth: For people who maintain a normal and nutritious intake of whole foods, there's absolutely no need to depend upon extra vitamins and mineral supplementation. There are virtually no studies proving vitamins and supplements to be of any value in the general population. This includes studies such as the *Women's Health Initiative*, which followed more than 34,000 women for 15 years. Vitamins had no positive effect on their health. Vitamins account for somewhere between $10 and $20 billion dollars spent every year in the United States, and this amount is growing, all without a shred of evidence that there is any benefit at all for the vast majority of people.

The exception to this may apply to a few special groups. One group would include athletes who are on very restrictive unbalanced diets because of demanding weight loss programs, or who may have, for any reason, a very unbalanced diet at all; and who also may be missing some essential food groups, minerals or other micronutrients. This is not a healthy basis for living anyway. The other groups who could potentially benefit from medically prescribed supplements include pregnant women and children who are not eating a fully enough balanced diet to meet their special needs. Here is where medical consultation would be very valuable. Also menopausal and postmenopausal women should check with their medical practitioners about their own needs for additional calcium.

Let's look at supplements specifically as they relate to weight loss and/or fitness programs. In 2009, the Federal Drug Administration (FDA) issued a warning and recalled an entire line of products that were sold as dietary supplements, which were marketed for weight loss, selective fat burning, energy enhancement, low carb diet aids, and to promote water weight loss. The FDA recall warned that they had received reports of severe illnesses, including 23 reports of serious health problems ranging from jaundice, which is the skin turning yellow from liver failure along with elevated liver enzymes, which can signal serious liver injury. One report of liver failure required a liver transplant and there was also one report of death due to liver failure. At least one of these reports was documented in a person taking only the recommended dose on the label, not an overdose. There were other reports of seizures; cardiovascular disorders; and something called rhabdomyolysis, which is the death of skeletal muscle, and which in itself can lead to other serious and even fatal complications including kidney failure.

The FDA recall included a line of 14 products from 1 company, some of which had names that included phrases such as "natural" and "caffeine free." These names designed to make the customers feel safer, because they were allegedly more natural. Many of the hundreds of other products out there used language in their sales pitches that tout ways to lose weight quickly and easily, employing what they called fat-burning supplements—in other words, lots of gain with no pain. I think we've all had our fill of the commercials on TV touting supplements and vitamins and all sorts of products with promises to make us bigger, thinner, stronger, more vital, and healthier. They offer us the opportunity to spend money on products with questionable ingredients to allegedly improve our health. Those ads often target children and pregnant women. Some go so far as to say their protein supplement is like human mother's milk—only better. They're ridiculous.

Let's look at another myth: Well, it's natural, so it must be healthy. Wrong! Some of the most potent poisons on Earth are natural, including: Belladonna Alkaloids—belladonna means "beautiful woman" because once these drugs used to dilate the pupils and make the eyes look large and mysteriously blacker. They can be very toxic in the wrong use or the wrong dose. Botulinum toxin, which milligram for milligram, is the most potent poison on Earth—is currently used in Botox. Also lifesaving, naturally-occurring drugs such as digitalis from purple foxglove can reverse heart failure; but in an overdose, can kill even a normal patient who has no heart disease at all. Even insulin, which is normally a lifesaving drug for diabetics, can be dangerous or lethal if it's taken in the wrong dose. The key word here is dose: the proper amount, in the right time, for the right person. When we're evaluating supplements, just as any other drugs, don't fall into the trap of thinking that natural means safe. Or worse, that if some is good, more is better. More may be very dangerous; dose counts.

Let's go from the myth that more is better, to another widely held myth: Athletes need large amounts of protein to increase muscle mass and strength, often taken in the forms of artificial supplements. Let's start by first defining the protein needs for the average person and then for someone who wants to build new muscle and increase their strength. Then we'll look to see what the science tells us about the needs for and the safety of protein supplements.

There are a lot of authors, doctors, and sports experts who suggest that high protein diets and protein supplements are necessary; and yet it's hard to find scientific evidence that proves this to be true. How big is the issue, and how biased might the profit motive influence the sellers? Sales of protein supplements in the United States are approaching $3 billion per year. This is big business. These products are sold with the promise of turning us ordinary humans into sculpted, ripped athletic gods and goddesses, with very little effort to become that way.

This is an especially tempting sales pitch to teens and young adults. In a 2005 study in the journal *Pediatrics*, the official journal of the *American Academy of Pediatrics*, investigators found that a large group buyers of these products were in the 12–18 year old range. More than 50 years ago, I was one of those skinny teenagers with baby giraffe legs, which I still have. The only help I had back then was something like the Charles atlas ads in comic books, promising to make me bigger with what we now call isometric exercises. Few if any supplements were on the market back then, because that was fortunate for me because I would have been one of those kids tempted by the idea of quick fixes to get huge muscles. Let's look at the science.

There are several facts about human physiology that get in the way of any kind of recommendations for very high protein intake. The key question is knowing how fast amino acids can be absorbed from the intestinal tract. Remember, the amino acids basic building blocks of proteins, and these amino acids are how these supplements generally supply the protein. Another question is how fast can the liver break down excess proteins and produce urea to get rid of the excess nitrogen, and stave off toxicity? Well, very high protein diets, in ranges such as 200–400 grams per day, which many supplement sellers suggest, probably exceed the liver's capacity to get rid of the excess urea nitrogen. One large review article concluded that it's dangerous when protein exceeds more than 35% of total caloric intake; this can lead to hyperaminoacidemia, which is too many amino acids in the blood; hyperammonemia, too much ammonia in the blood from the breakdown of the protein; hyperinsulinemia, too much insulin; as well as nausea and diarrhea. In some cases deaths have also been reported from all of these conditions.

To achieve balance you should look at 2 things: (1) the absolute amount of protein in grams per day; and (2) the absolute maximum recommendations, which is roughly one pound per gram per day of the body weight maximum—about 175 grams for a 175 pound person. And about 25% of total caloric intake, which would be 125 grams per day of protein if you ate the average of 2000 calories, or 4 calories per gram of protein. In this country we generally don't think in terms of grams, but all the nutritional information for a defined portion on the food labels and websites is stated in grams, so that should be fairly easy in determining amounts. You can also calculate your protein needs in grams by taking your body weight in pounds and multiplying it by 0.4. The ideal American male at 154 pounds, for him this would be around 60 grams. For a heavy duty athlete with high energy output and muscle building goals it could go up to about 1 gram per pound of body weight per day maximum. But no more, if anything I would err on the side of a little less—154 grams in our example, but in my opinion that would still be high. Remember, the body thrives on moderation, and in this case the moderation refers to the total daily protein intake. Here again dose matters.

Some other thoughts: The hype out there around protein today can still sound very promising—supposedly you can lose weight quickly, get a fast energy lift, build muscles, even boost the immune system so you won't get sick. Some ads go so far as to claim that protein supplements will deter the aging process. In other words: one giant quick fix for everyone.

In the July 2010 Consumer Reports it was published an evaluation of protein supplements. This is well worth reviewing for more detail. Basically this study used independent labs to investigate 15 different popular protein supplements. In addition, they did a survey of government papers on the subject and interviewed a wide range of health, nutrition, and sports experts. The key finding was that most people get sufficient protein in their regular diets already and that supplements offer very little if any benefits in addition. One product *Consumer Reports* tested recommended a dose amounting what amounted to 176 grams of protein dissolved in enough milk to add another 33 grams. That's 209 grams alone and is pushing the edge of safety. In addition, most people get another 82 grams of protein in their regular diet. When you add those supplemental 209 grams from the protein drinks to the average 82 grams, you're now already up to nearly 300 grams of protein. Which is way more than needed and already above the possible toxic levels, as I just discussed.

Let's move on from the issue of dose. How about the issue of content purity and safety? Apparently all the drinks that Consumer Reports tested had at least one sample containing one or more contaminants: arsenic, cadmium, lead, mercury. All these metals all have toxic effects on several organs in the body. *Consumer Reports* pointed out that the presence of cadmium is especially disturbing because it can specifically damage the kidneys. Remember that kidney damage is one of the risks of taking in too much protein in the first place; getting rid of the body's cadmium can take as long as 20 years to excrete just half the accumulated metal. For diabetics especially—of which we have millions in the U.S., and millions more who are heading in that direction but who have not yet been diagnosed—kidney disease is part of the diabetes problem itself; so diabetics certainly would not want to add more damage with even more protein or heavy metal accumulation.

For the vegetarian and vegan athlete there are all kinds of delicious ways to combine tofu, whole grains, and beans to make complete proteins for the body. Maintaining a balanced diet, including adequate calcium and protein is a bit more challenging for vegetarians when fish, poultry, meat, and dairy are not in the regular diet. For those athletes, I would highly recommend working with a nutritionist to ensure a proper balance.

Now a word about other risks: Protein excess also causes increased calcium excretion from bones. Long term use can also increase the risk of developing osteoporosis in both men, women, and younger people as well. While the supplement industry still argues that there is no upper limit of safety for protein if you balance your diet, most nutritionists and scientists disagree. And so do I. there is an upper limit for protein intake and your body knows it.

If you really don't need these supplements, and since there are real dangers to their use and overuse, what about the issue of comparable cost? Consumer Reports estimates that half a chicken breast with 27 grams of protein cost about 62 cents; and 3 8-ounce glasses of fat free milk, about 23 grams of protein cost about 60 cents; 3 scrambled eggs, 20 grams, about 46 cents. Compare this to 25 grams of protein in a scoop of one popular protein powder at about $1.61, or nearly 3 times the cost. You can meet your daily requirements for protein, and then some, in a safer, tastier, and cheaper way just by eating whole foods.

Let's look at another popular myth, around one very popular supplement, creatine. The myth is that creatine enhances growth promoting substances, enhances energy production, and increases the synthesis of muscle proteins.

Currently this myth approaches the level of gospel among bodybuilders. Creatine is among the most widely advertised and widely used of all the muscle building and performance enhancing supplements. Creatine is a naturally occurring molecule; it's found in human organs, muscles, and body fluids. It chemically combines with phosphate molecules to form something called phosphocreatine, which is a high-energy phosphate, and is active in the anaerobic phase of muscular contraction. This is one of the most widely sold supplements, especially among bodybuilders. It's vitally important that we first look at whether there might be harmful effects and secondly, whether it works at all.

Warnings on the label that come with this supplement include, weight gain, gastrointestinal upset, muscle cramps, dizziness, diarrhea, heat intolerance, dehydration, fever, reduced blood volume, and electrolyte imbalances. That's just for starters. Then there are some other possible risks, especially for diabetics on medication as well as individuals on diuretics, because creatine can increase the risks of dehydration and electrolyte disturbances— something I talked about that problem in the lecture on hydration. Creatine also may be a problem for the millions of people who take statins for high cholesterol, because creatine can increase cholesterol-lowering effects, which means interfering with dosage calculations. Taking caffeine, ephedra, and creatine together can also increase the risk of a number of other serious adverse effects. Creatine is not an innocuous substance just because it exists in nature.

Does creatine work? There are a few very small studies suggesting that that in short-duration, high-intensity sports, creatine might increase performance. But a large survey of the majority of the scientific literature did not confirm this. In 1999, a review article by Graham and Hatton, which you can find in our bibliography, a study from all around the world spanning over 33 years, from 1966–1999, the researchers found that the increased levels of creatine in the muscle might allow for the buildup of stores of phosphocreatine, which I mentioned earlier, and which could lead to extra energy in the form of adenosine triphosphate, or ATP, which is the final pathway for energy release in our cells. But, beyond this theoretical advantage, they were unable to show actual performance improvement with high-quality research.

Now, you could probably find almost any position you want to find if you scour the literature enough. If you really want to take creatine, it is easy to find a paper here and there to support its safety and its value. And you can find the opposite as well: Creatine is useless as well as potentially dangerous. But, when you look at the sum of studies which measured the important parameters of effort and endurance; endurance during isotonic exercises, that is the exercises that shorten the muscle such as a pull up or barbell curl; strength in isotonic exercises; total isometric force; and performance measured on ergometers there seem to be an equal number of results showing some positive results as well as showing no effect at all. But if you look at studies on athletes in their actual performance in the field away from the lab, there is even less evidence of any effect. Any benefit at all seems to be limited to very short-duration, very high-intensity efforts at the extreme edge of the energy envelope.

The authors of this very extensive Graham/Hatton study concluded that creatine is not useful in endurance sports and because creatine products are not controlled as closely as pharmaceuticals, these authors were also concerned about impurities and dose problems, just as we were about protein supplements, the very same concern we had with protein supplements themselves. Also there's no evidence that creatine improves performance in older people or women. The authors felt that in the light of marginal safety for any benefit coupled with any long-term safety, they didn't recommend using it. It is not a banned substance for professional or Olympic sports, but nonetheless there seems to be more folklore than real scientific data supporting its use, which makes me think of the word "myth"—remind yourself again that anecdotes from your muscle-building friends are just that, anecdotes not data. If a person is spending a lot of money and time on supplements, they have a vested interest in their own perception that the supplement is helping them.

Let's go on to another highly touted supplement. Myth: Quercetin is the new miracle substance that will allow us to reach higher performance levels, even without extra training. Now quercetin is a flavonoid compound, one of many found in nature that often have some antioxidant properties, as well as anti-inflammatory properties. Those are good things. It can be found in apple skins, berries, red wine, black tea, and some leafy vegetables. Because it has been shown as a possibly potent performance enhancer in mice, it has gotten the attention of human athletes as well. But, let's not make the jump from mouse to man too quickly. Is it a myth or not?

Let's see where the science is right now. In mouse experiments in the laboratory, investigators found some increase in markers of mitochondrial biogenesis, the energy powerhouse in cells. They speculated that this could have implications for human endurance, but before you run out to buy Quercetin supplements, let's look at some more data, this time a little higher up the evolutionary ladder than mice. In an early human study researchers compared elite male cyclists in a double-blind, randomized, crossover study which included a 30 kilometer time trial taking either twice daily doses of antioxidant supplements of vitamins with Quercetin for 6 weeks, or antioxidant supplements without Quercetin for 6 weeks and a control group who took nothing. Those who took the Quercetin increased their high-intensity time trial performance by increasing their power output. But a placebo also improved their performance. And there are an increasingly large number of studies in humans which show no effect for those taking Quercetin, including one study of ultra extreme 100-mile races—that's nearly 4 marathons! This study showed no improvement at all, on Quercetin.

The University of Georgia professor, Kirk J. Cureton, who ran some of these studies said that "There were simply no differences" between the Quercetin and the placebo group. He felt that this supplement may just not be effective in humans as in mice, which is often the case.

Are there any supplements that I do like? If I had to pick my number one favorite in the whole field, it would be fish oil. These preparations over and over again have been found to be healthy, and promote the rebalancing of some very unhealthy ratios in our modern diet—ratios of substances in these oils called DHA and EPA. There is an overwhelming body of evidence that most people in the Western world would benefit in many ways from the addition of about 1000 milligrams of fish oils per day. But our subject here is the relationship between nutritional supplements and fitness. So other than leading to a healthier life, there is no evidence that fish oils will improve athletic performance.

Let's move on to another myth: Sports and energy drinks are a safe and cost effective way to improve performance and maintain hydration.

First, as always, we need to make sure we have our definitions correct. The terms sports drink and energy drinks are often used interchangeably, and are not truly interchangeable. In general, sports drinks refer to those which are designed to maintain optimal hydration, and which may also contain carbohydrates and some electrolytes. They should not contain any stimulants. Energy drinks are similar to sports drinks, but also contain stimulants such as caffeine with the idea that they may boost performance.

Many sports drinks are merely water with some added sugar and flavor, and then artificial food dyes as well. In some cases added sodium and potassium to replace sweat losses. Why do we need to buy them at all, when most cost many times more than premium gas for your car? One of the most popular drinks costs $5 a quart. That's $20 a gallon! I can take tap water and add the juice of a couple of delicious lemons and a few teaspoons of sugar and get the same benefit, at much lower cost and more purity. At least I will know exactly what is in my drink. My take is that these drinks are a very, very expensive way to do what you can do on your own with every bit as much success. Try making your own with water, fruit juice, some sugar and salt.

Start out lighter on the sugar, try it, and then tweak the amounts to suit your tastes and your needs. Again, err on the side of moderation.

Energy drinks: Here is where it gets trickier. The advertising point is that these drinks escalate from replacement of lost water, sugar, and electrolytes, to adding some alleged power and performance boosters, which for one thing may have no proven benefit, while at the same time escalating some dangers. Most doctors and scientists today agree that the occasional energy drink may do no harm in selective athletes; but you have to be careful with other groups such as children, diabetics, and people with underlying cardiovascular diseases, or with anyone over doing it. The big issue is that these drinks may have an over-abundance of caffeine and sugar as well as a number of synthetic and herbal stimulants, which may be printed on the label. Most mask the fact that they are, in many cases, just sources of still more caffeine or caffeine-like drugs. These include maté and guarana. Other drinks contain ephedra, which is in Ma Huang, and pseudoephedrine, have been associated with serious complications. Many contain the amino acid, taurine, sometimes in very large doses. A number of review articles that neither benefit nor health risks occur with these drinks, but the same reviewers also noted that the amounts of guarana, taurine, and ginseng found in popular energy drinks may be well below the doses expected to deliver any benefits. More evidence of receiving nothing at great cost.

The side effects of large doses many of the stimulants in energy drinks can cause at a minimum, irritability, restlessness, insomnia, headaches, and nausea. Higher on the dangerous side, they can cause increases in blood pressure and a racing pulse. This kind of cardiac response in turn ups the risk for heart rhythm disturbances, which in themselves can trigger very dangerous cardiac events including chest pain, heart attacks, and cardiac arrest. Epileptic seizures have also been reported. Many trainers are cautious about the increased irritability, because it can cause nervousness just when the athlete needs to be calm and focused.

With all these considerable risks, are there any benefits? Especially, do they improve performance? Probably not on both counts. Because the manufacturers call these dietary supplements, they are not controlled by the FDA. The manufacturers can make claims that the drinks improve performance or mental acuity with no science of their own to back this up, and no evidence about their safety.

Before we end, here are a few things to remember: (1) When it comes to supplements, natural does not mean safe. (2) With few exceptions people who maintain a normal and nutritious diet do not need vitamin and mineral supplementation. (3) Active individuals with sufficient protein in their diets do not need protein supplements. (4) Studies involving humans show little evidence to support the performance-boosting claims of supplements such as Creatine, Quercetin, or most of the proprietary compounds. (5) If you do choose to take a supplement, beware of possible contaminants and limit your dosage based on established daily requirements and existing medical conditions. And (6) consider using your own recipe for a sports drink, at lower cost and greater purity without the hidden dangers.

I keep coming back to some basic truths. First and foremost, it's not nice to fool Mother Nature. Next you rarely get something for nothing, while nutritious whole foods and hard work will stand the test of time. Shortcuts will usually get you lost.

Thank you.

Can You Get Too Much of a Good Thing?
Lecture 5

Overdoing exercise and/or extreme dieting are trends that seem to be on the rise, and the consequences can be severe. Children, young adults, and older adults can all suffer from too much of a good thing.

Myth: You can never be too thin.

Extreme diets tend to fall into one or more of several categories. At the top of the list are starvation diets; these are often touted as cleansing or detoxification diets. They usually include some form of drastic caloric restriction, along with the use of laxatives. But the body has finely tuned mechanisms for detoxification of virtually every cell and organ, and you will only upset these mechanisms by going to extremes.

Some very low-calorie start-up diets can work under the right circumstances. Generally, these are short term, carefully structured, and monitored by medical and nutritional experts to avoid starvation symptoms. In the end, what ultimately gets rid of unwanted fat is a long-term, mild reduction in calories; a healthy diet of fresh, whole foods; and a sensible, lifelong fitness program.

In extreme diets, malnutrition and dehydration are definite risks. Measurements on extremely low-calorie diets show that about half the weight loss is fat and the other half is from lean tissues, such as muscle. On more moderate diets, fat loss represents about three-quarters of the lost weight and protein or muscle, only about a quarter.

Myth: You can never exercise too much.

While serious eating disorders tend to be much more prevalent in women, activity disorders occur more often in men. Some common symptoms of **exercise addiction** include frequent injuries; frequent illnesses, caused by running down the body's immune system; and the inability to complete exercise routines that were once doable, probably again, from running down the body with insufficient time for rest and repair. This is a complex disorder that should be addressed by an experienced therapist or physician.

We know that the body improves its fitness through mild levels of injury, followed by repair and rebuilding. That's why heavy weight training is generally limited to every other day for major muscle groups. In the syndrome of excess, there is more than mild injury and insufficient time for repair.

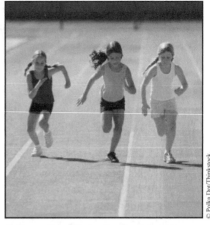

Orthopedic and sports physicians have found no benefit to extreme, regimented exercise programs for children.

How can you tell the normal pain of exertion from the bad pain of overdoing it? The most familiar discomfort you feel during exercise is "the burn." This pain tends to feel superficial and evenly spread over and in the muscle mass. Compare that sensation with localized, sharp pain in the knee or ankle. Usually, this pain worsens at each impact. This kind of pain is an injury and is generally caused by inflammation. Your body is telling you to stop and apply **RICE**—rest, ice, compression, and elevation.

Myth: Starting rigorous exercise programs in very early childhood will prepare your kids for a top-flight athletic life and achievement.
Many parents are lured into getting their children into sports programs by the idea that it will make them candidates for athletic scholarships or even sports careers later in life. But orthopedic and sports physicians at some of the nation's top pediatric hospitals tell us that there is no research to support the idea that such extreme or regimented programs will make children better coordinated or stronger.

If your child loves gymnastics class, you should definitely support that interest, but don't start picturing Mary Lou Retton; you're setting yourself up for disappointment, placing your child under too much pressure, and replacing the joy of the sport with competition.

Childhood is a critical developmental stage for bones, ligaments, tendons, and joints, and injuries at a young age can cause severe and irreversible growth problems. Children can get overuse injuries just as adults can, but they might never get over the effects. There is also the issue of burnout. Pushing youngsters into sports and activities that they don't want to do may turn them off from any sort of body movement. ■

Eating Disorders in Teenagers

Eating disorders are not uncommon in one particular group of weight losers: teenagers. Weight, as it reflects upon self-image, is an obsession in the U.S. especially among teen girls. About 15% of women in general have some eating obsession. About 35% of adolescent girls see themselves as overweight, and about 60% are trying to lose weight. There are a few telltale signs from the *American Psychiatric Association* that can alert us to these conditions in our children or friends. Some warning signs of bulimia might include:

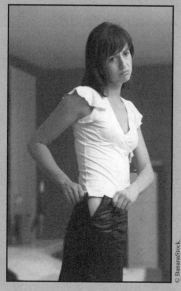

© BananaStock.

- Extreme preoccupation about weight, often unjustified.

- Alternating strict dieting with binge eating.

- Disappearing from sight after meals.

- Unwarranted and frequent use of laxatives or diuretics.

- Excessive aerobic exercising and training.

Unhealthy Weight in Sports

Certain sports activities tend to be more conducive to this excess focus on weight, for example ballet, gymnastics, running, and swimming. For young men, this dance between weight loss and maintaining muscle strength is as serious and potentially dangerous as anorexia and bulimia is for women.

The Yo-Yo problem: Many high school and college men play more than one sport, often as many as three. These athletes may go back and forth in weight gain and loss to accomodate different sports such as increasing weight in the fall for football, where every pound of muscle and fat is treasured on the field; and then slimming down in the winter when they switch to wrestling, where fat and excess muscle weight may disqualify you.

The Female Athlete Triad problem: In recent years there has been a recognition of a triad of conditions showing up more and more in young women athletes. A sign is an obsession with physical exercise, in intensity, frequency, and duration. It seems that excessive exercise causes a reduction in estrogen levels, which leads to **amenorrhea**. The osteoporosis probably results from a combination of a low calcium diet as well as the low estrogens.

Dairy is often left out because of the fat issue, so teen girls are getting lower doses of calcium and Vitamin D, which then worsens the risk for osteoporosis. Body weight itself influences bone density; pathologically low weight does not stimulate stronger bone formation; so restrictive low calorie diets can lead to osteoporosis all by itself. One of the most common first signs of the onset of this triad is the occurrence of fractures in young women athletes.

Today, sports oversight organizations such as the NCAA and others are trying to establish criteria and restrictions surrounding weight loss; and establish certification for each athlete's minimum healthy weight. One promising approach has been to determine a healthy weight and healthy state of hydration early in the season before competition begins. This is a good start at controlling the dangerous excesses in what is supposed to be sport, not a life and death struggle.

Lessons from the Lecture

(1) When it comes to supplements, natural does not mean safe.

(2) With few exceptions, people who maintain a normal and nutritious diet do not need vitamin and mineral supplementation.

(3) Active individuals with sufficient protein in their diets do not need protein supplements.

(4) Studies involving humans show little evidence to support the performance-boosting claims of supplements such as creatine, quercetin, or most of the proprietary compounds.

(5) If you do choose to take a supplement, beware of possible contaminants and limit your dosage based on established daily requirements and existing medical conditions.

(6) Consider using your own recipe for a sports drink, at lower cost and greater purity without the hidden dangers.

Important Terms

amenorrhea: the cessation of menstrual periods.

anorexia nervosa: a general term for an extreme psychological disorder that involves disturbances in eating behavior. In anorexia the patient refuses to maintain what we would define as a normal body weight. They actually see their bodies in a totally different light than we would see them.

bulimia: eating disorder where the person often engages in episodes of binge-eating followed by forced vomiting and laxatives to purge the food. Many of these people add on hours of aerobic exercise to burn off calories as well.

exercise addiction: when people are not able to not exercise—even in the face of severe injuries, of truly bad weather, physical exhaustion or illness—they just can't stop. Some common symptoms include frequent injuries; frequent illnesses, from running down the body's immune system; and the inability to complete exercise routines that were once doable, probably again from running down the body with insufficient time for rest and repair.

RICE: acronym for attending to an injury meaning rest, ice, compression, and elevation.

Suggested Reading

Crowley and Lodge. *Younger Next Year.*

Hartmann. *Walking Your Blues Away.*

Kessler. *The End of Overeating: Taking.*

Powers and Thompson. *The Exercise Balance.*

Web MD. "Teen Girls' Health: Understanding Eating Disorders in Teens."

Questions to Consider

1. What is the difference between anorexia nervosa and bulimia, and which of these, if either, is more common in male athletes?

2. Define exercise addiction. What is its relationship to eating disorders?

Can You Get Too Much of a Good Thing?
Lecture 5—Transcript

Welcome back. In this lecture we're going to look at the myth that says, "If a little is good, more is better." In other lectures in this series on food and fitness, I've talked about finding your own balanced path to health and wellness.

Today, I'd like to talk about what happens when we get unbalanced and go overboard in the belief that if a little is good, more is better in any direction. There are several disturbing and increasing trends in the numbers of people who are both over-exercising and over-dieting. This is also what has been defined as an "addiction" to exercise coupled with severe eating disorders. Overdoing exercise and/or extreme dieting can happen at any age; and the consequences can be severe across the board. Children, young adults, as well as older adults can all suffer from too much of a good thing.

First, let's look at this myth as it applies to extreme diets. Wallis Simpson, The Duchess of Windsor, once said "You can never be too rich or too thin." Well, I don't know about the "too rich" part, but speaking as a doctor, I'd say that the idea that you can never be too thin is a very dangerous myth. Let me give you a brief clinical history: A 28 year old woman had a history of anorexia nervosa diagnosed by her family physician when she was 24. She had been steadily losing weight, going from 130 pounds (at 5'7") down to 95 pounds when her family finally intervened. She had a long history of fad diets and was constantly miserable about her body image and her looks. She underwent psychotherapy and seemed to be doing well over the next few years, recovering her weight to about 110 pounds without any apparent further problems.

She moved away from home to take a new job in another city at age 27. Six months later after she left, her parents were called and notified that she was dead on arrival at a local emergency room near her apartment. A friend had found her after not being able to reach her by phone for several days.

Police found her medicine chest and kitchen cabinets containing several forms of diet pills, many kinds of vitamins, and 2 different kinds of over-the-counter emetics (drugs used to induce vomiting). She had a supply of disposable saline enemas as well as laxatives. There was evidence of recent vomiting as well as a large supply of high fat foods such as fried chicken, potato chips, and ice cream in her refrigerator, freezer, and pantry. There was also a lot of half-eaten food. The police investigation also found that she had belonged to a local gym, and was known to spend several hours there almost every day or evening, making extensive use of cardio equipment, as well as a rubber suit and the sauna.

At autopsy her body weighed 80 pounds, and she appeared to have suffered extensive muscle atrophy. Blood toxicology screening and tissue samples showed no evidence of any drugs or other toxic substances. Her organs were normal except for some early fatty changes in the liver (suggesting chronic starvation) and an abnormally dilated colon (suggesting over-use of enemas and laxatives). The pathologist called the cause of death heart failure secondary to starvation and severe electrolyte imbalance from anorexia nervosa and bulimia nervosa. We'll talk about the 2 of those in a minute.

This is a story so common, that by today's standards—except for the families and friends of these patients—it's hardly noticed. And although most of the patients are virtually anonymous, I could show a long list of celebrities, both living and dead, with similar histories. Extreme diets tend to fall into one or more of several categories. (And here when I use the term "diets," I am speaking about ways to lose weight rather than my preferred healthy and balanced approach to the original Greek meaning of *diaita*, "a way to live.")

Right at the top of the list are starvation diets in one form or another, and these are often touted as cleansing diets, as well as detoxification diets. They've been around for ages, and usually include some form of drastic caloric restriction along with juices and supplements, and a cleansing regimen that can include oral laxatives, both natural or chemical—or approaching from the other end, so-called "cleansing enemas" of various substances from plain water to coffee. In a word, avoid all these diets like the plague. They are nonsense, they don't work, and they're dangerous.

As to the enemas, and detoxification in general: Again, there is not a shred of evidence that they work, and they can be exceedingly—even lethally—

dangerous. As a surgeon, I've had the sad job of operating on a patient who had a colon perforation—causing a potentially deadly fecal contamination of their abdominal cavity—from a badly performed detox enema. I had to give this poor soul a temporary colostomy which she kept for months until healing was complete and until I could safely go back and put her together again. These detox techniques are completely unnecessary and ineffective. They should be abandoned totally. The colon does a fantastic job of cleaning itself because it's designed with muscle function to move the feces along in only one direction: down and out. Repeated enemas not only move the fecal content in the wrong direction, but can lead to completely over-stretched muscles, leaving the colon flabby and ineffective—like an over-inflated balloon. Our bodies have evolved over millions of years to our present state where it has wonderful and finely tuned mechanisms of detoxification for virtually every cell and organ in our body. You will only upset these mechanisms by going to extremes.

Also, in extreme diets, malnutrition is a definite risk. In other words, entering a phase of nutritional imbalance or "starvation" is what we risk. We can also become dehydrated, upsetting the balance of our electrolytes and other minerals as well. Any of the severe diets get risky after a few weeks. Going for a loss of more than a pound or so a week is unrealistic in the long term, and probably unhealthy.

Remind yourself that the statistics for people who do go on starvation diets or drastic diets are dismal. As we saw in another lecture, the vast majority will be back to their higher weight within a year. Measurements on extremely low calorie diets show that about half the weight loss is fat and the other half is from lean tissues such as muscle. In the more moderate diets, fat loss is about three-quarters of the lost weight and protein or muscle loss only about a quarter—much more desirable. Remember, too, that resting muscle burns more calories than resting fat. You want to preserve your muscle (the lean mass) and minimize the fat. You do this by continuing to exercise as well as moderating your diet. There are a number of very low-calorie startup diets that can work under the right circumstances. Generally, these are short-term, carefully structured, and monitored by medical and nutritional experts to avoid starvation symptoms. For these I suggest seeking the consultation and guidance of a registered dietitian or doctor who specializes in these diets.

In the end, what ultimately gets rid of the unwanted and unhealthy fat is a long-term mild reduction in calories, coupled with a healthy diet of fresh whole foods, along with a sensible long-term and enjoyable fitness program. Since optimal health is a lifelong endeavor, it's wiser to get off any of the very restrictive diets as soon as possible, and go back to translating "diet" as a way of living rather than as a way of just losing weight. Make your goals attainable and not dramatic.

There is one group of people who are often overly-focused on weight loss and concern me most: teenagers. Remember the case history I used in the beginning of this lecture; the same pattern is all too common among teen girls. Unfortunately, eating disorders in teens are not uncommon. Doctors all too often see the combination of patients forcing themselves to vomit along with the abuse of laxatives and unhealthy eating patterns. This is a serious health problem.

One cause of this problem is that weight, as it reflects upon self-image, is an obsession in the United States, especially among teen girls. Here are a few alarming statistics: About 15% of women in general have some eating obsession; about 35% of adolescent girls see themselves as overweight; and about 60% of adolescent girls are trying to lose weight. In the area of eating disorders among both teen boys and girls, 90% are girls. The boys are more concerned about the muscularity of their bodies and more often overreach with regard to over-exercising and supplementation more than diet.

Let's review a few definitions before we move on. Anorexia nervosa is a term for an extreme psychological disorder that involves disturbances in eating behavior. In anorexia the person refuses to maintain what we would define as a normal body weight. They actually see their bodies in a totally different light than we would see them. With bulimia, they often engages in episodes of binge eating followed by forced vomiting and laxatives to purge the food. Many bulimics add on hours of aerobic exercise to burn off calories as well.

From a practical point of view, there are a few telltale signs *The American Psychiatric Association* tells us that can alert us to these conditions. Some warning signs of bulimia might include: extreme preoccupation about weight, often unjustified; alternating strict dieting with binge eating; disappearing from sight after meals, presumably to induce vomiting in private; unwarranted and frequent use of laxatives or diuretics; excessive aerobic exercising and training. In addition, certain sports and activities tend to be more conducive to this excess focus on weight. Ballet and gymnastics are 2 of them. Also, running and swimming can over-emphasize the value of a thin physique. Wrestling, which I'll discuss in a minute, can overemphasize both thinness as well as muscle gain.

I had an experience in college rowing which illustrates exactly what I'm talking about. At the time it seemed just a normal part of the sport. Lightweight crews must average 155 pounds at 6 PM the night before the race, and no single oarsman can weigh more than 160 pounds. As in wrestling, a single man or the entire crew might be disqualified, so the weigh-in was critical. My normal weight at that time was about 155 pounds—which was right on the nose—but I still had to lose 11 pounds every week so that I and one other of the oarsman could help average down the crew's total weight. We happened to have a very big group of oarsmen in my boat, many whom would normally weigh about 170 pounds when they were already fit and lean. To get down to the 160 pound maximum, we all suffered days of starvation (lettuce sandwiches stands out in my mind) and dehydration followed by only an overnight grace period to rehydrate and to eat. And I had to do the same, even though I was already quite thin. There were hours of sweating in rubber suits just before the weigh-in. It was unhealthy and it was dangerous. And much like weight loss in wrestling, everyone did it. For young men, this dance between weight loss and maintaining muscle strength is as serious and potentially dangerous as anorexia and bulimia is for women.

There is another serious concern in young men who participate in the sport of wrestling. If a wrestler fails to make weight, he is out of the competition. In this sport, there have been documented deaths from pre-match dehydration. Fortunately today, oversight organizations such as the NCAA and others are trying to establish criteria and restrictions surrounding weight loss, and establish certification for each athlete's minimum healthy weight. One promising approach has been to determine each athlete's healthy weight and healthy state of hydration early in the season before the competition begins. This takes into account such things as proper hydration by analyzing the urine. Then body-fat is measured, with a minimum healthy fat level for men being no lower than 7% and 12% for women. There are also maximum levels of weight loss allowed per week. This is really a good starting point at controlling dangerous excesses in what is supposed to be a sport, not a life and death struggle. The fact that young athletes have died trying to make weight for high school and college sports is outrageous.

But that's not the whole story. There's also the yo-yo problem. Many high school and college men and women play more than 1 sport, often as many as 3. If they play football in the fall (where every pound of their muscle and fat is treasured on the field) and then switch to wrestling in the winter (where fat and excessive muscle weight can disqualify them), they get caught in an impossible health dilemma. Unfortunately, these teens and young adults are often in a serious state of denial about this issue just at a time in their lives when communication between parents and children may be under stress anyway.

These lectures are not the forum for the diagnosis and treatment of these disorders, it's only a place to bring it to your awareness. This is a serious medical matter and a threat to both mental and physical health. I highly recommend individual expert consultation with your physician if you want to learn more.

Let's look at another area for concern: the recently documented phenomenon called "the female athlete triad." This triad is a serious problem. In recent years there has been a medical recognition of this triad of conditions showing up more and more in young women athletes. The 3 in this triad are: eating disorders of various kinds which result in energy deficits with subsequent cessation of menstrual periods (amenorrhea) and osteoporosis (low bone mass). One additional sign is an obsession with physical exercise, in intensity, frequency, and duration. What seems to happen is that the excessive exercise causes a reduction in estrogen levels, which leads to amenorrhea (the loss of the menstrual periods). The osteoporosis probably results from a combination of a low calcium diet as well as the low estrogens. And body weight itself influences bone density. Pathologically low weight does not stimulate stronger bone formation, so restrictively low calorie diets can lead to osteoporosis all by itself.

If we look at the extreme cases, the eating disorders tend to be exactly the ones we've already discussed: anorexia, bulimia, and extreme dietary restriction. Dairy is also often left out because of the fat issue, so these young women are getting lower doses of calcium and Vitamin D, which then worsens the risk for osteoporosis. It's also well-established that osteoporosis in the young is a risk factor for osteoporosis in late adulthood, so this is an important factor to address because it also has lifelong implications.

One of the most common first signs of the onset of this triad is the occurrence of fractures in young women athletes. For example, young ballet dancers can develop stress fractures in their feet, ankles, and legs with what would be considered very little force in an otherwise normal person. The key here is vigilance by the athlete, her trainer, her parents. They all need to be alert for signs of extreme diets, marked weight loss, cessation of menstrual cycles, and fractures. If there is any question about this, I urge you to seek professional guidance and get a consultation before the damage is done. Bone density measurement is easy, it's safe, it's accurate, and it can help prevent factures which could at worst result in impaired limb or joint function and also end a promising athletic career. There are several resources for this list in our bibliography.

So far we have been dealing with the very dangerous myth that you can never be too thin. Here's another myth I want to address: that you can never exercise too much. This involves actual addiction to exercise. Some have called it "exercise disorder" or "activity disorder." It doesn't matter how we label it. There is a segment of the population who are absolutely not able to not exercise. This is true even in the face of severe injuries, of truly bad weather, of physical exhaustion, or illness. They just cannot stop. And they often couple this extreme compulsion with unhealthy dietary habits such as fasting, bulimia, diet pills, laxatives, or diuretics. Their professional and personal lives can suffer as well when individuals focus too intensely on exercise, creating an unbalanced lifestyle.

Again, an interesting observation is that while the serious eating disorders tend to be much more prevalent in women (especially young women), these serious activity disorders occur more often in men. Most people who are into a more balanced level of fitness—even some very high level athletes—

generally look forward to their down time as that of rest, relaxation, and repair. At the opposite extreme end of the spectrum, some individuals are actually ill at ease and anxious when they are not exercising. They get a sense of achievement and self-worth from being stressed by the exercise, and training outdoors in the bad weather, and the deprivation of comfort, whether that comes from not eating or over-exercising.

Some common symptoms of exercise addiction include very frequent injuries, frequent illnesses from running down the body's immune system, and an inability to complete exercise routines that were once doable— probably again from running down the body with insufficient time for rest and repair. We know that the body improves its fitness by mild levels of injury followed by repair and rebuilding. That's why heavy weight training is generally limited to every other day for major muscle groups. In the syndrome of excess, there is often more than mild injury along with insufficient time for repair. And of course, over time, performance will also begin to decline instead of improving. This is a very complex disorder, and requires an experienced and skilled therapist, physician, or other expert in the field. In general, it's not something that a family member or friend can handle alone. They need well trained help.

Before we leave the subject of too much of a good thing, I want to get back to "listening to your body." I come back to this idea in different places in this series of lectures on nutrition and fitness for a very good reason: It's a good rule. People often ask me just how they can tell the difference from, for example, different kinds of pain. What is the difference between normal or good pain of exertion and the bad pain of overdoing it?

While I can't give you hard and fast rules because it's very subjective, there are some guidelines that might help. Let's start with the most familiar discomfort, "the burn." Most of us know that as we reach our limits on almost any activity, we begin to feel what we describe as a burning pain spreading though the muscles in use. It tends to feel superficial (on the surface) and very evenly spread over and in the muscle mass. It's not generally worsened by impact (such as in running) but it's more a steady state. This is the body response to reaching the limits of the metabolic needs for your muscles—

running out of steam. And pushing this to its limit can be useful, especially if you allow enough recovery time for rest and repair.

Compare this with, let's say, a specific pain in your knee or your ankle which is localized and sharp, tending to feel as if it's right in the joint. Usually it's worst at each impact, say, again, if you're running. This kind of pain is an injury, and is generally caused by inflammation. It's a signal. Your body is telling you, "Stop! I'm injured." You might be able to continue by altering your gait or your balance or some other adjustment, but in these cases while you protect one joint, you might be overstressing another joint. Saving the knee and injuring the hip, for example (what some call "pushing through the pain"). The body says stop, so stop. It's R.I.C.E. time: rest, ice, compression, and elevation. (Let me just add that the C, compression, is not one of my favorites because it can be easily overdone if you're not careful.)

What else can you listen to in your body? Well, for me, it's often necessary to know when my body is telling me I am a little over-fatigued. That trap is one I know I have to avoid and push myself to get some movement—maybe not a hardcore high-intensity interval training workout, perhaps just a brisk walk up some hills—something to get me out of the lethargy and the excuse phase and into some body movement that will usually make me feel better when I'm done.

On the other hand, you might wake up with a fever, or a sore throat, or the headache/muscle aches and pains that signal the beginning of a viral illness. Listen to and heed those symptoms as well. Of all the things you could easily measure, such as pulse, blood pressure, and so on, your body temperature will give you the best indicator of a real illness. If you have a fever, this too might be the real sign that says, "Skip the exercise today." It might be just the time to roll over and go back to bed. You will not do your body any good in pushing through the illness any more than pushing through the inflammatory pain of an injured ankle. Listen to your body. It knows what it needs.

Finally, I want to touch on another related topic. Myth: starting rigorous exercise programs in very early childhood will prepare your kids for a top flight athletic life and achievement. The myth is about the current fad of extreme exercise for younger children and toddlers. I want to talk about this even though it might not bear directly on nutrition. Because in a word, nothing should change in how you feed your kids relative to what they are doing for exercise. All children of every age should be fed a well rounded nutritious diet of whole foods, rich in fruits and vegetables, with lots of choice and variety. Period.

As to when you may be pushing the envelope too far in terms of training, endurance, strength, and getting your little ones ready for the 2040 Olympics or the Major Leagues, let's just agree that it's totally nuts that we even have to have this discussion at all. But unfortunately, we do. Many parents are being lured into getting their children into sports programs even as young as toddlers—3 or 4 years old—with the idea that it will make them better athletes, better competitors, candidates for athletic scholarships, or even a career in professional sports. Orthopedic and sports physicians at the nation's top pediatric hospitals tell us that there's absolutely no scientific data to back up any ideas that your children will be better coordinated or stronger from extreme and regimented programs. If your kid loves running around in the gymnastics class, great. Go for it. But don't start envisioning gold medals; you're setting yourself up for disappointment, and you're placing your child under way too much pressure and stress—both physical and psychological. And you'll certainly take the joy out of it once you force them into that competitive mode.

The same applies to many of the organized sports that can so easily go from a good day of running round with friends on a soccer field to screaming parent-spectators yelling at well-meaning referees. It can easily morph into not such a pretty picture. And the downside has long-term consequences that are extremely dangerous. First of all, kids' bones, ligaments, tendons, and joints are in a very critical developmental stage. Injuries at this young age can cause severe and often irreversible growth problems, with limb shortening and chronic disabilities or deformities. Children can get overuse injuries just as adults can, but their bodies might never get over the effects.

Secondly, there's the issue of burn-out. Pushing youngsters into sports and activities they may not want to do, or may not want to continue is more than counterproductive. You might end up with a jaded child who doesn't want any part in any body movement. A child who's allowed to select his own or her own activities—ones where they have an interest or a possibly innate talent—will blossom and thrive on their own. Again: you can't fool Mother Nature, especially with the little ones in your care. And there's no need to. If you have ever tried to keep up with the physical movements of a toddler, you'll know without question that they don't need any programs to keep them moving. They will run and jump and climb far beyond your physical ability to keep up with them. That's why playgrounds have benches—for you, not for the kids. Let the little ones do what comes naturally. Intense competition and pumping iron should not be in their world, and for very good reasons.

In summary: (1) There are real dangers in pushing the envelope too far whether it's in the form of weight loss diets or muscle gain diets, as well as the physical fitness envelope that borders on compulsive activities. They are dangerous and insidious, so keep alert. (2) Moderation serves most of us very well, and we need to recognize when we're exceeding safe and healthy levels. Each of us can and needs to find our own personal sweet spot. (3) As to children, they have no business being out there on the edges of the envelope. Keep them moving and happy, but keep them safe. They will find the ways that serve them best. Again, we can follow their lead to find the joy in our own body movement.

Thank you.

Going To Extremes—The Smart Way
Lecture 6

This lecture focuses on individuals who push the edges of the envelope, those who explore and endure very high or low altitudes or extremes of heat or cold. Those who push their bodies to extreme limits need a different focus from those of us whose exertion and environment are more controlled and a bit more moderate.

Myth: Humans can adapt to virtually all the Earth's environments if given enough time, enough training, and basic equipment.
In any extreme environment—low altitude or high, hot or cold—it's essential to have a proper respect for the elements. Few of us will ever be faced with the challenge of altitudes approaching 26,000 feet, but thousands of people go from sea level to, say, 11,000 feet just to go skiing or hiking. A common ailment called **acute mountain sickness** can affect those who live low and ski or hike at high altitudes. Symptoms include headache, insomnia, dizziness, dehydration, and fatigue. The best prevention and cure for mountain sickness is to stay hydrated.

Going from a high to a very low altitude is not as much of a problem for humans. The lowest points on dry Earth vary from –282 feet in Death Valley to about –1,400 feet at the Dead Sea. The real problems in those places would be the extremes of dry heat and the threat of dehydration.

Myth: Humans are the weakest and the slowest of animals, who depend upon their brains rather than their brawn for success and survival.
Mankind certainly is at the top of the evolutionary ladder as far as brain development is concerned, and that level of intelligence has made up for a relative lack of strength and speed. But that's not the whole story. Against nearly every animal on Earth, if the human can select the distance, he or she will have a good chance to win the race. Not many animals can run for 26 miles, as we can, and even fewer can regulate their pace without changing their gait. On the other hand, it's not just any person who can get out of

bed tomorrow morning and run a 26-mile race. Extreme events, such as marathons and mountain-climbing, require special preparation.

We get all our energy at the cellular level by using carbohydrates circulating in the blood in glucose. We store excess glucose in muscles, the liver, and other organs as a complex molecule called **glycogen**. In general, your muscles and liver can store enough glycogen for a moderate to high level of exercise and activities. When you begin to run out of backup glycogen, performance can degrade and fatigue sets in. Humans can switch over to burning fat when they run out of glycogen, but this is a relatively inefficient process, and performance suffers. Glycogen stored in the muscles can be used only for muscle contraction and not shared with other body organs; the liver glycogen, on the other hand, can be converted and released into the bloodstream to benefit every other organ.

As a way to top off the total tank of glycogen in the liver and muscles to ensure the maximum available amount for exertion, many endurance athletes have latched onto **carbohydrate loading.** Some recent studies have found

Lessons from the Lecture

(1) For extreme places you may want to go—high or low, hot or cold, wet or dry—it's all about the preparation. Ask yourself which mistake would you rather make? To take too much food and water and shelter in your backpack or get caught without enough?

(2) For most short-duration recreational activities and brief high-intensity efforts, carbohydrate loading will do nothing for your performance and might have some down side effects.

(3) If you choose to carbohydrate load at all, do so moderately under supervision of a sports medicine expert, especially if you are diabetic.

(4) Even with carbohydrate loading, you will probably need extra supplemental carbohydrates during the event.

that elevated muscle glycogen before exertion delays fatigue by about 20% in endurance events lasting more than 90 minutes, but final answers after decades of study are not yet in. There are also some downside risks to carbohydrate loading, such as weight gain, which may lead to decreased performance; intestinal gas and bloating or diarrhea, which can influence performance due to dehydration; and problems caused by wide swings in blood sugar from using complex carbohydrates instead of simple sugars.

Most experts who believe in carbohydrate loading suggest increasing the carbs to about 50–60% of total calories in the week prior to the event and scaling back the training level in the last few days before the event. Topping off the glycogen stores in the liver and muscles may be a good thing, but overdoing it will probably serve no purpose because there is only so much glycogen the body can store. ■

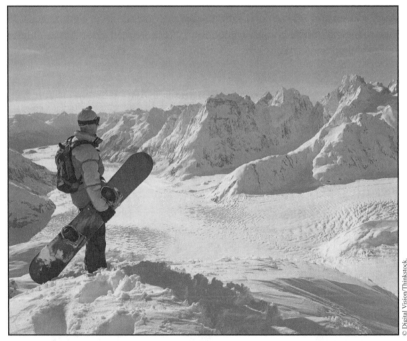

In extreme environments—low or high altitude, hot or cold temperatures—it's essential to be prepared for the elements.

acute mountain sickness: ailment due to the change from low- or sea-level altitudes to altitudes over 8000 feet. It usually involves symptoms such as headache, insomnia, dizziness, dehydration, and fatigue. It tends to go away in a day or 2 with some rest and acclimatization, and the best prevention and cure for this is to stay hydrated.

carbohydrate loading: plan to increase the amount of stored glycogen in the body to use as energy reserves, often used by endurance or extreme athletes.

glycogen: complex molecules comprised of glucose and stored in muscles, liver, and other organs.

Suggested Reading

Clark. *Growing Old is Not for Sissies II*:

Galloway. *Marathon*.

Isserman and Weaver. *Fallen Giants*.

Ryan. *Sports Nutrition for Endurance Athletes*.

Questions to Consider

1. Define the Death Zone. What is its significance in acclimatization for high-altitude events?

2. What is insensible water loss? What is the effect of altitude on insensible water loss and how can you ameliorate its effects?

Going to Extremes—The Smart Way
Lecture 6—Transcript

Welcome back. We'll start today by looking our first myth in this lecture on going to extremes: Humans can adapt to virtually all the Earth's environments if given enough time, enough training, and basic equipment. But first, let me begin with a story. In the spring of 1978, I was the doctor on a trek in Nepal to the famous mountain called Annapurna. This was the first of the 8000 meter Himalayan peaks to be climbed, by Maurice Herzog in 1950. I was 10 when he first climbed it, and it was a mountain I had always wanted to see ever since. One day at the end of the trip, I was very lucky to be stranded at a remote grass airstrip there for 6 hours, waiting for a small plane (which it turned out was 6 hours late every day). I say I was lucky because I was stranded with Tenzing Norgay, the famous Sherpa who was the first man to summit Mount Everest with Edmond Hillary in 1953, and a personal hero of mine ever since.

We had a lots of time to talk, and during the course of the conversation, Tenzing told me he thought Everest could be climbed without oxygen. I didn't want to be rude or contradict the man who had been there, but I said to him it seemed physiologically impossible without oxygen, because once you climbed into the so-called "Death Zone" above 8000 meters (26,000 feet), the body starts dying slowly but surely, and no amount of acclimatization is possible. Above 26,000, feet no living organism can exist for very long. For humans, survival might be measured in just days.

Tenzing was of course very polite, but he was insistent. He said, "I don't mean the way I climbed Everest, with multiple camps above 26,000 feet. You're right. Not with Sherpas and hundreds of bottles of oxygen and support teams and equipment and several days to go the next 3000 feet to the summit and down again. But perhaps someone in fantastic shape who could go alone in a lightning strike right up and right down again without support, and in a short enough time so that he could survive without oxygen." Tenzing looked very wistful and said, " I think it can be done."

I shrugged, and I thought he was probably wrong, but I thanked him for his conversation. I was so thrilled just to have had the chance to spend this time with him that I didn't give it a second thought until just a few months later when Reinhold Messner, an Italian-born mountaineer, became the first human to climb Mount Everest without supplemental oxygen—a feat he would do again 2 years later, this time climbing solo, just as Tenzing said. Messner later became the first human to climb all 14 of the world's 8000 meter mountains.

Reinhold Messner is an example of the kind of athlete I want to focus on today: individuals who push the edges of the envelope, who achieve record-breaking feats, who explore and endure very high or very low altitudes, or extremes of heat or cold, people who can exert themselves for very long durations. This is where we humans push our body to not only extreme limits, but possibly very dangerous ones as well. Here's where we might need a different focus from those of us whose exertion and environment are more controlled and a bit more moderate.

When we consider what some men and women have accomplished at these extreme edges of the envelope, sometimes there seems to be no limit to what a dedicated human can do if they're trained and motivated. From my perspective, I still believe that the reality is in many cases that there are limits. For example it is still thought to be impossible to acclimatize to altitudes above 26,000 feet. Period. This is still called the Death Zone and likely will always be. No creature on Earth has been found to survive there for any prolonged period of time. Messner just bypassed the physiology by being so strong and well-trained and determined, that he could make that ascent up and down again before the mountain killed him. But he would not have been able to stay at altitude for a longer duration no matter how fit he was; it is inherent in our physiology.

Let's discuss altitude in a bit more depth. I mentioned the infamous Death Zone, which is roughly above 26,000 feet or 8000 meters. Few of us will ever be faced with that kind of challenge. But thousands of us go from sea level to some high altitudes, for example, just to go skiing. It's not uncommon to fly from sea level and be skiing at 11,000 feet within 24 hours, or to be hiking at that same altitude or higher; I've done that myself many, many times. For those of us who do this, there is usually very little risk compared to Himalayan mountaineers who go twice as high on a regular basis. But there is a well-known ailment called "acute mountain sickness," which is common among people who live at low altitudes and ski or hike at much higher elevations. It's common enough around 8000 feet where many Rocky Mountain ski resorts are located. Acute mountain sickness usually involves symptoms such as headache, insomnia, dizziness, dehydration, and fatigue. It tends to go away in a day or 2 with some rest and acclimatization. The best prevention and cure for this is to stay hydrated. I'll get to that more in a minute.

In these lectures we've been more interested in how extreme exertions and extreme environments impact our food and water intake than on our conditioning and acclimatization. For now, the important point is not so much a discussion of the partial pressure of oxygen at various altitudes, or of the serious illnesses such as high altitude pulmonary edema where the lungs fill with water, or cerebral edema where the brain swells dangerously (both of which can kill you in hours), but rather the most pressing issues of hydration plus nutrition and conditioning. When you're exerting yourself even moderately, let's say hard downhill skiing at 10,000 feet, you'll be losing a lot of water as you breathe, and even more insidiously from sweating, even if there are no visible signs of sweat, because the water evaporates so quickly from your body in the cold, dry mountain air. You definitely need to markedly increase your usual intake of water to make up for the insensible losses. For example, when you go from sea level to 6000 feet your water loss simply from breathing doubles; at 10,000 feet this insensible water loss actually triples.

And in the extreme conditions, say when you are out for a prolonged period of time in very cold weather and at high altitude, don't make the common mistake of thinking you can always rely on eating that lovely white snow around you to rehydrate; you can't. Snow is mostly air, so 12 inches of snow will have only 1 or 2 inches of water in it. It will take more of your body heat and energy to melt enough snow in your mouth than you'll get back in hydration from the snow you are eating. At altitude, you need either to carry all your water—which is not practical for a long expedition—or have a source of heat to melt the snow, such a portable stove powered by bottled gas or solid fuel.

And remember, you'll also burn many more calories in the extra physical exertion that high altitude requires, as well as just keeping the body warm at very low ambient temperatures. You need to carry light-weight, high-energy sources of calories with you in the form of preparations designed for high altitude expeditions—power bars, freeze dried meals. Even if it's just a day of skiing or cross-country snow shoeing in the backcountry, you're going to need some help.

And one added piece of advice: Never go out into the relative wilderness (especially in the mountains)—even for a day's outing at high altitude or wintry weather—without being prepared to stay and survive overnight. You never know when you might get lost, or simply sprain an ankle, or get caught in an unexpected snowstorm. I've had that experience happen to me in the middle of July in the Colorado Rockies. Without the extra equipment and food in my backpack, it might have been a lot more serious than an adventure to tell my grandkids. This may mean toting a heavier backpack, but it could save yours or someone else's life.

Now let's consider going from very high to very low, which is not generally as much of a problem for humans. The lowest points on dry earth vary from minus 282 feet in Death Valley to roughly 1200 feet below sea level in the Dead Sea in the Middle East. So here we're talking about relatively small changes in atmospheric pressure in those places. The real concern in those areas would be the extremes of dry heat and the threat of dehydration. And here, you won't have the issue of whether you can melt snow in your mouth. No snow, no water. Everything you drink will have to be carried in. So hydration is the real issue, and this is a matter of planning—period. Your life or death from dehydration will be your responsibility. It's all about preparation. Food and nutrition becomes secondary in these low, hot, dry environments; it's all about the water—a subject I discuss at length in the lecture on hydration. There have been a number of investigations about the effects on cardiac and pulmonary function at extremely low altitudes such as the Dead Sea, but these have been inconclusive and sometimes contradictory. At the moment, I think the issue is that of dehydration and staying safe rather than peak performance.

In any extreme environment—high or low, hot or cold—it's essential to have proper respect for the elements. While I was with Tenzing Norgay I asked him how it felt to be the man who conquered Everest. And Tenzing said, "No, sir. No one conquers Everest. If you are very, very lucky, you will be permitted to walk upon her back and survive." Tenzing's humility is a good example for any of us who are considering extreme activities, especially outdoors.

On the other hand, the fact remains that humans can achieve some pretty remarkable physical feats, which is why I'd like to address another myth that gives our species too little credit. This widely held myth says humans are the weakest and the slowest of animals who depend upon their brains rather than their brawn for success and survival. There is a kernel of truth in this, as there is in most myths. Most scientists agree that humankind is at the top of the evolutionary ladder as far as brain development is concerned, and that level of intelligence has made up for our relative lack of strength and speed. But that's not the whole story. For example, humans actually can outrun almost any animal, but only as long as the human chooses the distance. So if you were being run down by a cheetah, which can run nearly 60 miles an hour, you would become dinner. But in a more theoretical vein, you can run 26 miles faster than the cheetah can. In fact, against nearly every animal on Earth, if the human can select the distance, he or she will have a good chance to win the race. Not many animals can run for 26 miles as we can, and even fewer can regulate their pace without changing their gait. For instance, a horse must go from a walk, to a trot, to a cantor or gallop as it increases its speed, so it is forced to change its efficiency. Humans can choose the most efficient gait and still regulate speed appropriate to the distance. And most of us can think ahead to plan the gait and the timing.

On the other hand, it's not just any person who can get out of bed tomorrow morning and run a 26-mile race. Extreme events such as marathons and extreme mountain-climbing require special preparation. Anyone who trains hard for such events is probably going to continually look for ways to improve their performance during the event itself. One method many endurance athletes have latched onto is carbohydrate loading. But are the benefits of carbohydrate loading just a myth? Certainly the stories about carbohydrate loading sometimes attains mythical status. Depending on the person you're talking to, the myth of carbo-loading might be worded in 1 or 2 very different ways. The first version of the myth is that extreme carbohydrate loading is an important regimen for endurance athletes, and is absolutely the key to success in long, hard endurance contests. The second version of the myth is that carbo-loading is of no value to the endurance athlete and is dangerous to your health. And I could go on to write a plausible lecture to fit either side of the argument.

For this lecture I'll have to refer to the "debate" rather than the "myth," because the answer isn't obvious. In essence, the debate revolves around whether or not loading up with carbohydrates before a major endurance event will improve performance. Let's consider sports that require high energy output for more than 90 minutes. For instance, runners of marathon races use up extraordinary amounts of energy. That's 26 miles 385 yards to be exact. That means running for more than 2 hours for even the fastest runners, and it can take over 8 hours or more for some of the slower runners. The same applies to a triathlon. The Ironman triathlete swims 2.4 miles, then bikes 112 miles, then finishes by running the 26 plus miles. The very fastest of these athletes will still put in more than 8 hours of grueling endurance and effort. We're talking about a whole different level of exertion here.

Long-distance endurance sports such as marathon running and triathlon competitions have moved from the sport of just a few diehard athletes, as it was when I was young, to encompassing literally tens of thousands of competitors at huge events worldwide. In the 2009, the New York City marathon had about 44,000 runners finish the race. And as more and more people participate in extreme events, the question of the value of carbohydrate loading only becomes more relevant. This is no longer a minor issue among a small group of athletes. The debate on this issue is very old. Over 30 years ago, an article appeared in the *British Journal of Sports Medicine*. It was titled "Glycogen loading: advantages but possible disadvantages." The debate has raged on ever since.

Before we get into the evidence for and against carbo-loading, let's start by looking at the basic physiology of energy demand and energy production. Remember, we get all our energy at the cellular level by using carbohydrates circulating in the blood in the form of simple sugar (glucose). We store excess (or reserves) of glucose in our muscles, in the liver, and in other organs as a complex molecule called glycogen. In general, your muscles and your liver can store enough glycogen for moderate- to high-level exercise and activities which last less than about 90 minutes—a very rough figure. After that point, performance can degrade and fatigue sets in because you begin to run out of the backup glycogen (and therefore out of sufficient glucose). Humans can switch over to burning fat when they run out of glycogen, but this is a relatively inefficient process, and performance really suffers.

Let me be clear when distinguishing between workout programs aimed at burning fat and workout programs aimed at attaining peak performance. When you are in an extreme exertion mode, you want to use carbohydrates for fuel, and not fat. Remember that the glycogen stored in your muscles can be used only for muscle contraction, and cannot be shared with other organs such as your brain, which also needs glucose. And by the way, the brain and the heart have no glucose reserves at all. They need second-to-second replenishment from circulating glucose in the blood. The liver glycogen, on the other hand, can be converted and released into the bloodstream to benefit every other organ including the brain and the muscles as well. The theory is that carbohydrate loading might be able to top off the total tank of glycogen (in the liver and muscles) to assure the maximum output for your exertion. If it doesn't, you are going to need a supplement during your exertion in the form of glucose containing foods or beverages.

Okay, so that's a quick overview of the physiology. Now let's look at whether carbohydrate loading will in fact improve athletic performance. First, it's important to remember again, that for most recreational activity, your body can and does use its existing energy stores for fuel. It's pretty well agreed that carbohydrate loading is not necessary for short events and events requiring very high intensity burst-efforts such as sprinting or weightlifting; and carbohydrate loading will not improve performance in those arenas. With these short duration events, generally under an hour, researchers found little or no effect using techniques that elevated pre-exercise muscle glycogen contents above normal resting levels for athletes. Similarly, they found no effect in moderate-intensity exertions (like running or biking) from 60 up to about 90 minutes. They found substantial useful quantities of glycogen still remaining in the muscles at the end of a moderate exercise period.

Now let's consider long and to extreme endurance events—more than an hour or 2 in duration. If we don't need carbo-loading for the short-term, high-intensity efforts, what's the current science regarding its use in the long-duration events? The earlier more extreme versions of carbohydrate loading have just not been supported by science. In those early days (in the 1970s and '80s), carbo-loading started about one week before the big event. But, at that time the athletes would first make their carbohydrate intake less than half of their total calories. Then they would maintain a high level of exertion to deplete the rest of the stores of glycogen, to theoretically make room for the carbo-loading. Then, about 3 or 4 days before the event, the athletes would increase the carbs way up to about 70% of calories. At the same time they would lower their daily training way back, to preserve these new glycogen stores until race day.

The idea was that under stress, the cells would go into emergency mode and make it possible to store even more glycogen than usual. It was a good theory. But did it work? Unfortunately there's not a lot of science to show that this extreme form of carbo-loading works any better than more moderate programs. There's not a scientific basis to back up the idea that really depleting glycogen stores primes the cells to overload with carbs later on. And, remember that not all athletes find carbo-loading beneficial. Many athletes still feel serious fatigue, or run into the famous "18-mile wall" in a marathon, where many totally run out of gas, even after carbo-loading.

To look at this, researchers tested 2 groups of high level cyclists. One group had a 3-day carbo-load, and the control group did not. Then they conducted 100 kilometer time trials (that's over 60 miles), which included several segments of very high-intensity sprinting as well.

In all of the aspects measured, there was no significant difference in the performance and the endurance between the carbo-loading group and the controls. This study suggested that carbo-loading did not improve performance. And there are some downside risks to carbo-loading as well. For example, many athletes gain water weight on high carbs, and this can decrease performance all by itself. Others get gastrointestinal gas and bloating, which can be very disconcerting during a race or other long-distance events. High carbs can cause serious diarrhea—another real danger which could influence your performance due to dehydration. Wide swings in blood sugar levels can also be a problem with carbo-loading—best diagnosed and treated by a physician. Using complex carbohydrates instead of simple sugars in advance of the event can help stave off these wider swings in blood sugar, yet there is no evidence that the complex carbs are any better than simple sugars during the event. Before you decide to carbo-load, you should get some professional advice from either a certified dietitian or your physician. This is especially true if you have any medical conditions, the most important of which would be diabetes. Diabetics compete at very high levels in many sports throughout the world, but their glycogen and nutrition in general should be managed with great care and great caution by a professional.

There are many other variables to consider in training, including the age and even gender. Women for some unexplained reason seem overall to get less benefit from carbo-loading than men. They might need more carbs than men, or they may just not get the benefit. Unfortunately, there is much less research available on women overall right now. Additionally because the body still has a maximum storage capability which no amount of loading will exceed, during your event, you will need an additional 30–60 grams of carbs per hour along the way; that's about 2–5 packets of sugar. Ultimately, in long distance and prolonged exertion events, you will still need even more carbs such as snack or an energy drink containing simple sugars in them. Most of the experts today who believe in carbo-loading at all suggest just increasing carbs to about 50–60% of total calories in the week prior to the event, and scaling back the training level in the last few days prior to the event.

Even at this extreme end of the exertion spectrum, it seems to me that some moderation will serve you well. Topping off the glycogen stores in your liver and muscles could be a good thing. Overdoing it will probably serve no purpose, since there is only so much glycogen the body can store. Finding that sweet spot is more difficult. If I were an ultra-marathon runner or an extreme athlete, I would put my training and nutrition into the hands of an experienced sports medicine specialist, and follow her advice. The science here is still in flux, and even in the world of controlled studies, there are legitimate differences of opinion among scientists.

Now let's talk about some new studies that have appeared on the horizon. Recently a group of British researchers studied some generally elderly, very, very high-level, life-long athletes. They looked only at men from British national or British Olympic teams in long-distance running or rowing. They also focused on men who had completed more than a 100 marathons. What they found was a little disturbing: About half of these older lifelong athletes showed heart muscle fibrosis (scarring) on magnetic resonance imaging (MRI). They were generally the ones who had trained the hardest for the most years in a group of already highly trained people. There have been some other studies around the world with similar findings, as well as a few animal studies. But the cause-and-effect is still a long way from being established, and these findings would only apply to a very tiny fraction of all endurance athletes.

But since this lecture deals with the extremes of exercise and endurance, it's only fair to include this new research as more information comes to light. We want to alert you to be vigilant if you are pushing the most extreme edges of the envelope. Remember that exercise in general is extremely good for overall health. In the case of brain function, there is nothing that could even come close to exercise for preventing things like cognitive decline. The same benefits apply to your heart, your blood pressure, and general life functions.

I want to end the discussion on carbo-loading with one story I love from the 1981 New York City Marathon. This is about the great marathon runner Alberto Salazar. Apparently the story goes that 2 days before the race, Salazar went into the Carnegie Delicatessen and ate a huge pastrami sandwich with a pound of meat—dripping with fat and full of protein. Two days later he won his second of 3 consecutive New York marathons and broke the record. I love that story because it goes against all the conventions for proper training. It brings us right back to the individualizing of our training methods and listening to our bodies.

In closing, let's keep several things in mind: (1) As to the extreme places you may want to go—high or low, hot or cold, wet or dry—it's all about the preparation. Ask which mistake you would rather make: To take too much food and water and shelter in your backpack, or get caught without enough? (2) For most short-duration recreational activities and brief high-intensity efforts, carbo-loading will do nothing for your performance, and might have some downside effects. (3) Even when we are talking about the long-duration events such as marathons and triathlons, there is still much debate and a lot of anecdotal evidence where there is yet to be strong science. (4) It's my opinion is that it's probably prudent, if you choose to carbo-load at all, to do so moderately under supervision of a sports medicine expert—especially if you are diabetic. (5) Keep in mind that even with carbo-loading, you will probably need supplemental extra carbohydrates over the course of the long-duration event. The amount will depend upon your particular body makeup, your gender, age, and conditioning, as well as the terrain, the altitude, and the temperature. One size definitely does not fit all, so you need to consult the latest recommendations for you. (6) On a final note, I'd look at the thoughts and beliefs we feed ourselves. Some recent studies with solid research support the idea that it highly beneficial in many ways for us to ease up on the self-criticism that we heap on ourselves; that if we can accept our foibles and our imperfections, we will find an easier and much more effective path to good health. This applies even when we undertake extreme challenges as well as for those of us who play on a more moderate scale of effort and danger. It's been shown that people who forgive themselves and have compassion for themselves suffer less in the way of depression, and are in general happier and more optimistic. (I'd bet they perform better as well, but that's just my opinion on that one.)

Our bodies have evolved into magnificent machines that in combination with our brains can take us to the most diverse places of any animal on Earth. We only have to take care of it and be prepared. Listen to your mother; listen to your body; take it easy on yourself; and enjoy the ride.

Thank you.

Glossary

acute mountain sickness: ailment due to the change from low- or sea-level altitudes to altitudes over 8000 feet. It usually involves symptoms such as headache, insomnia, dizziness, dehydration, and fatigue. It tends to go away in a day or 2 with some rest and acclimatization, and the best prevention and cure for this is to stay hydrated.

adenosine triphosphate (ATP): molecule found within cells that carries energy.

amenorrhea: the cessation of menstrual periods.

anorexia nervosa: a general term for an extreme psychological disorder that involves disturbances in eating behavior. In anorexia the patient refuses to maintain what we would define as a normal body weight. They actually see their bodies in a totally different light than we would see them.

body-mass index: The gold standard of population-based measurements of overweight. Take your weight in pounds, multiply it by 703, and divide by your height in inches squared; a BMI of less than 24.9 is considered normal weight, between 25 and 29.9 is overweight, and greater than 30 is obese.

bulimia: eating disorder where the person often engages in episodes of binge-eating followed by forced vomiting and laxatives to purge the food. Many of these people add on hours of aerobic exercise to burn off calories as well.

calorie: A unit of measure that estimates how much energy is metabolized.

carbohydrate loading: plan to increase the amount of stored glycogen in the body to use as energy reserves, often used by endurance or extreme athletes.

cardiac output: the volume of blood pumped on each beat of the heart.

complex carbohydrate: Groups of carbohydrates known as polysaccharides; they take longer to be broken down into their component parts than simple carbohydrates do and therefore are a healthier choice.

creatine: a naturally occurring molecule; found in human organs, muscles, and body fluids. It chemically combines with phosphate molecules to form something called phosphocreatine, which is a high-energy phosphate, and is active in the anaerobic phase of muscular contraction.

diuretic: something that stimulates increased urine output.

dynamic equilibrium: where fluids are shifting back and forth for redistribution to where they are needed at any specific time, and for maximum efficiency.

exercise addiction: when people are not able to not exercise—even in the face of severe injuries, of truly bad weather, physical exhaustion or illness—they just can't stop. Some common symptoms include frequent injuries; frequent illnesses, from running down the body's immune system; and the inability to complete exercise routines that were once do-able, probably again from running down the body with insufficient time for rest and repair.

fats: also known as lipids; the most energy dense of all the macronutrients, at 9 calories a gram. They are made up of carbon, hydrogen, and oxygen and function as an energy source, thermal insulator, hunger depressor, and vitamin carrier.

glycemic index: A measurement of how quickly blood sugar rises after the ingestion of a particular carbohydrate food.

glycogen: complex molecules comprised of glucose and stored in muscles, liver, and other organs.

healthy plate rule: a guideline to follow for healthier eating consisting of a plate that is half or more full with vegetables and fruit; a quarter or less with some lean meat such as fish, poultry, beans, nuts, tofu, or lean cheeses; and the rest complex carbohydrates such as grains or whole wheat bread.

internal milieu: term to describe the internal environment of cells.

interstitial space: the space between the cells. It holds about 10–12 quarts of water.

intracellular space: the water and salt inside your cells. This makes up about 25 quarts, a very large percent of the body's total water. Very critical in the management of cell function.

intravascular space: both blood cells and plasma inside our blood vessels, the most critical place for circulation, respiration, and oxygenation, delivery of energy containing compounds, and the removal of wastes.

obesity: Any body mass index of greater than 30. The 3 different types of obesity that have been defined are hypercellular, hypertrophic, and hyperplastic.

pre-workout meal: a light meal 1–2 hours before exercise consisting of about 200 calories, which is low in fat, moderate in proteins, and highest in complex carbohydrates.

protein: From the Greek word *proteios*, meaning "primary." Protein can be found in every tissue in the body; its main function is to build and repair tissue.

quercetin: a flavonoid compound, one of many found in nature that often have some antioxidant properties, as well as anti-inflammatory properties. It can be found in apple skins, berries, red wine, black tea, and some leafy vegetables.

RICE: Acronym for attending to an injury meaning Rest, Ice, Compression, and Elevation.

satiety level : the amount of food intake that will make you feel full.

Bibliography

General

Arria, Amelia M., and Mary Claire O'Brien. "The 'High' Risk of Energy Drinks." *JAMA* 305, no. 6 (2011): 600-601. Published online January 25, 2011. doi: 10.1001/jama.2011.109.

Benardot, Dan. "Timing of Energy and Fluid Intake: New Concepts for Weight Control and Hydration." *ACSM's Health & Fitness Journal* 11, no. 4 (July-August 2007): 13-19. doi: 10.1249/01.FIT.0000281226.23643.de

Bilsborough, S, and N. Mann. "A review of issues of dietary protein intake in humans." *International Journal of Sport Nutrition and Exercise Metabolism* 16, no. 2 (April 2006):129–52.

Bittman, Mark. *Food Matters: A Guide to Conscious Eating with More Than 75 Recipes.* New York: Simon & Schuster, 2008.

———. *How to Cook Everything: 2,000 Simple Recipes for Great Food.* Hoboken, NJ: Wiley Books, 2008.

Centers for Disease Control and Prevention. "U.S. Obesity Trends." http://www.cdc.gov/obesity/data/trends.html

Clark, Etta. *Growing Old Is Not for Sissies II: Portraits of Senior Athletes.* San Francisco, CA: Pomegranate Artbooks, 1995.

Consumer Reports Ratings Sports Drinks. http://www.consumerreports.org/cro/food/beverages/energy-drinks/energy-drinks-9-07/ratings/0709_drink_rate.htm

Crowley, Chris, and Henry Lodge. *Younger Next Year: Live Strong, Fit and Sexy until You're 80 and Beyond.* New York: Workman Publishing, 2007.

Galloway, Jeff. *Marathon: You Can Do It*. Bolinas, CA: Shelter Publications, 2010.

Hartmann, Thom. *Walking Your Blues Away: How to Heal the Mind and Create Emotional Well-Being*. Rochester, VT: Park Street Press, 2006.

Harvard Medical School. "Calories burned in 30 minutes for people of three different weights." Harvard Health Publications. http://www.health.harvard.edu/newsweek/Calories-burned-in-30-minutes-of-leisure-and-routine-activities.htm

Herbal Research Foundation. "Herbal Stimulants." http://www.herbs.org/greenpapers/stimulant.html

Hyman, Mark, and Mark Liponis. *Ultraprevention: The 6-Week Plan that Will Make You Healthy for Life*. New York: Scribner, 2003.

Isserman, Maurice, and Stewart Weaver. *Fallen Giants: A History of Himalayan Mountaineering from the Age of Empire to the Age of Extremes*. New Haven, CT: Yale University Press, 2010.

Kessler, David A. *The End of Overeating: Taking Control of the Insatiable American Appetite*. Emmaus, PA: Rodale Books, 2009.

Lehrer, Jonah. "The Truth Wears Off." *New Yorker*, December 13, 2010.

Mateljan, George. *The World's Healthiest Foods: Essential Guide for the Healthiest Way of Eating*. Seattle, WA: George Mateljan Foundation, 2007.

Mayo Clinic Recommendations for Energy Drinks.
http://www.mayoclinic.com/health/energy-drinks/AN01630

Mayo Clinic. "Caffeine Content for Coffee, Tea, Soda and More."
http://www.mayoclinic.com/health/caffeine/AN01211

"Nutrition and Athletic Performance." Joint Position Statement. *Medicine & Science in Sports & Exercise* 41, no. 3 (March 2009): 709-731. doi: 10.1249/MSS.0b013e31890eb86.

"Nutrition and Athletic Performance." *Medicine & Science in Sports & Exercise* 41, no. 3 (March 2009): 709–731. doi: 10.1249/MSS.0b013e31890eb86

Olshansky, S. Jay, Douglas J. Passaro, Ronald C. Hershow, et al. "A Potential Decline in Life Expectancy in the United States in the 21st Century." *New England Journal of Medicine* 352 (March 17, 2005): 1138–1145.

Pollan, Michael, *In Defense of Food: An Eater's Manifesto.* New York: Penguin Press, 2009.

Powers, Pauline, and Ron Thompson. *The Exercise Balance: What's Too Much, What's Too Little, and What's Just Right for You!* Carlsbad, CA: Gürze Books, 2007.

Robbins, John, and Dean Ornish. *The Food Revolution: How Your Diet Can Help Save Your Life and Our World.* Berkeley, CA: Conari Press, 2001.

Robbins, John. *Healthy at 100: How You Can—at Any Age—Dramatically Increase Your Life Span and Your Health Span.* New York: Ballantine Books, 2007.

Roizen, Michael F. and Mehmet Oz. *You Staying Young: The Owner's Manual for Extending Your Warranty.* New York: Free Press, 2007.

Ryan, Monique. *Sports Nutrition for Endurance Athletes.* Boulder, CO: Velo Press, 2007.

Stover, Beth, and Bob Murray. "Drink Up!: The Science of Hydration." *ACSM's Health & Fitness Journal* 11, no. 2 (March–April 2007): 7–12. DOI: 10.1249/01.FIT.0000262486.81937.4b.Taubes, Gary. *Good Calories, Bad Calories: Fats, Carbs and the Controversial Science of Diet and Health.* New York: Vintage Books, 2008.

Web MD. "Teen Girls' Health: Understanding Eating Disorders in Teens."
http://teens.webmd.com/understanding-eating-disorders-teens.

Websites/links

American Dietetic Association. "Sports, Cardiovascular and Wellness
Nutrition." http://www.scandpg.org

Consumer Reports Health.
http://www.consumerreports.org/health/home.htm

Harvard School of Public Health. "The Nutrition Source."
http://www.hsph.harvard.edu/nutritionsource

National Eating Disorders Association.
http://www.nationaleatingdisorders.org

University of California–Berkeley. "Wellness Letter."
http://wwww.wellnessletter.com

USDA Center for Nutrition Policy and Promotion. "Dietary Guidelines for
Americans." http://www.cnpp.usda.gov/dietaryguidelines.htm

U.S. Food and Nutrition Information Center. http://www.nutrition.gov

Notes

Notes

DATE DUE